Diabetes
COOKBOOK

Mini lamb roast with
red wine gravy, page 176

Diabetes
COOKBOOK

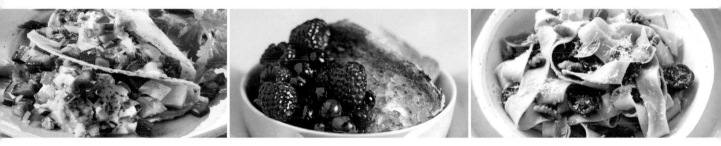

More than 140 RECIPES
to Balance Your Blood Sugar

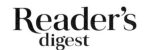

Reader's
digest

The Reader's Digest Association, Inc.
New York, NY/Montreal

CONTENTS

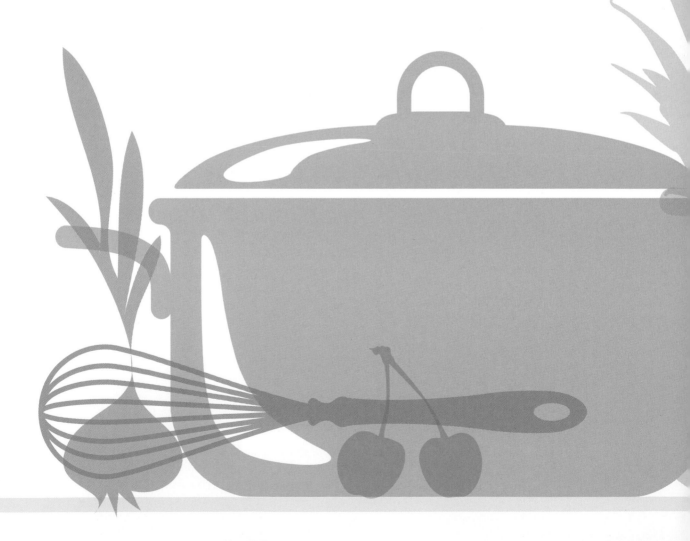

INTRODUCTION

O ver the last decade, dietary advice for diabetes has undergone a bit of a revolution. This new thinking is part of a larger, more intuitive approach to managing diabetes. Diabetes is a condition in which your blood glucose levels are abnormally high. The aim of diabetes management is to keep blood glucose within an optimal range and prevent complications. With guidance from your diabetes team, this can be achieved through healthy eating, exercise, maintaining a healthy weight and medication, if required. People with diabetes should eat a diet that is low in saturated fat, no added sugar or salt, and plenty of fruits and vegetables. The right amount of carbohydrate foods, such as bread, potatoes, cereals, pasta and rice, is also important. Here is an overview of the key nutrients a person with diabetes should consume.

A NOTE ABOUT THE RECIPES
The recipes in this book are suitable for people with diabetes. Each recipe includes a thorough analysis of key nutrients, including calories, protein, fat (including saturated fat), carbohydrates (including sugar), fiber and sodium. Note that foods that are included in the serving suggestions or that are optional are not included in the nutritional analysis.

sugar

People with diabetes don't need to avoid sugar completely. Sugar can be included as jam on some high-fiber toast or honey on oats as part of a healthy meal. However, candy or soft drinks that contain mostly added sugar are not recommended unless for treatment of hypoglycemia (low blood glucose). Unlike sugar, artificial sweeteners, such as aspartame, do not affect blood glucose levels. Use them to sweeten foods after cooking or to add to drinks. If you regularly use artificial sweeteners, choose a variety of different types.

carbohydrates

The body's main source of energy is carbohydrate. Everyone's carbohydrate needs are different but these foods should provide approximately half of your food intake for the day.

Carbohydrate foods contain either added sugar or natural sugars. Carbohydrates that contain natural sugars include fruit and fruit products, milk and yogurt, grain and cereal products and starchy vegetables such as potatoes, sweet potatoes and corn. Added sugars are found in candies, soft drinks, chocolate, cakes and cookies.

Carbohydrate foods are broken down in the body into sugars and, finally, to glucose. These foods have the most impact on your blood glucose levels of any foods. Eating carbohydrate foods regularly throughout the day will fuel your body and also help to keep blood glucose levels steady. Whole-grain cereals and breads, sweet potatoes and rolled oats are particularly recommended. Your dietitian can advise you how much carbohydrate to eat and when.

fatty foods

Fats are a class of organic chemicals that scientists refer to as fatty acids. When digested, they produce nearly double the energy of the same amount of carbohydrate or protein. Fat is only a problem when you eat too much of it and especially of the less healthy type. Fat molecules are stored in your body and this can result in weight gain. Carrying too much weight can impair the action of insulin and therefore cause higher than normal blood glucose levels. The build-up of fat-related molecules in your bloodstream is bad for your heart and circulatory system.

As with carbohydrates, it is wrong to say that all forms of fat are bad. There are three main types of fats, and two of these offer health benefits, so consider adding them to your diet—in appropriate amounts.

Fats that are in liquid form at room temperature (primarily plant oils, such as corn, olive or canola oil) are split into two categories: polyunsaturated and monounsaturated. Both have benefits, but the latter are best for you. There is evidence that monounsaturated fat raises your HDL (good) cholesterol, which is important for people with diabetes because they have an increased risk of heart disease. Monounsaturated fat also has been shown to reduce insulin resistance.

Then there are the fish oils, or omega-3 fatty acids. These are essential to the body and are found in oily fish such as tuna, salmon, herring, mackerel, trout and sardines. Research shows that eating oily fish as part of a healthy lifestyle can help to lower the risks of heart disease. You should consume oily fish at least twice a week.

The type of fat that is least healthy for you is known as saturated fat and is solid at room temperature. Primarily, this means butter, cheese and the fat on meat. It also includes coconut and palm oil. Saturated fat has the most detrimental effect on your blood cholesterol, which in turn makes you more prone to certain diseases. It is therefore best to avoid or limit the amount of saturated fats you eat.

Trans fatty acids are a result of how some fats and oils are processed. They are generally found in manufactured foods such as cookies and cakes. Studies show that these fats act like saturated fats and can raise your blood cholesterol levels, so it is important to avoid foods that show "hydro-genated vegetable oils" at the top of the ingredients list.

salt

Eating too much salt is linked with high blood pressure, so it is advisable to cut down on salt intake in order to reduce the risk of heart disease. According to the government's Dietary Guidelines for Americans, 2010, people with diabetes should only consume 1,500 mg of salt per day. Most Americans consume more than twice that amount. If you consume a lot of processed meals and snacks, it is very likely that you are taking in far more salt than you need.

How to cut down on salt
• Measure the amount of salt you add in cooking and gradually reduce the amount. You will soon get used to eating less salt.
• Avoid adding salt at the table.
• Experiment with dried and fresh herbs and freshly ground spices instead.
• Replace salt-rich foods with low-salt products.
• For varied flavors, try lime juice, balsamic vinegar and chili sauce.
• Read food labels carefully: Salt may appear as sodium, sodium chloride, bicarbonate of soda or monosodium glutamate.
• Cut down on salty foods such as chips, salted nuts, savory crackers and pretzels.
• Salted and smoked foods such as bacon, sausages, smoked fish, some canned fish and other processed convenience foods are often loaded with salt.
• Whenever possible, eat fresh fish, meats and vegetables; they contain only a small amount of naturally occurring salt.

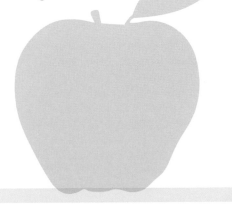

breakfast & brunch

chapter 1

fruit *smoothie*

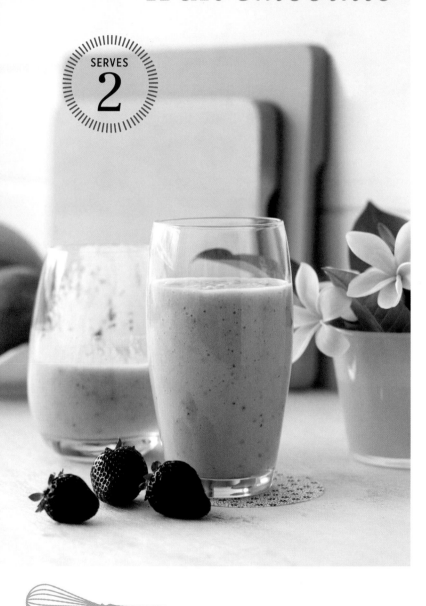

SERVES 2

SERVES 2   PREPARATION 5 MINUTES
COOKING NONE

1 cup (250 ml) low-fat milk
1 ripe banana or mango,
   peeled and cut into chunks
1/4 cup (50 g) fresh or frozen
   blueberries or strawberries
1 teaspoon (5 ml) honey, or to taste

1 Combine all the ingredients in a
   blender and blend until smooth.
2 Pour into two glasses and serve.

OTHER IDEAS

+ *Replace the milk with soy, almond or
  rice milk. Alternatively, use low-fat
  fruit-flavored yogurt, or a mix of fruit
  juice and plain yogurt.*
+ *You can use dried fruit (apricots,
  pitted prunes or dates), but you may
  need to soften them first by soaking
  or gently simmering them in water.*
+ *Add a pinch of spice, such as ground
  nutmeg, cinnamon or ginger.*
+ *For added nutrients, extra options
  include protein supplement powders,
  wheat germ, flaxseed, sunflower
  seeds and almonds, and soft nuts
  such as walnuts or pecans.*

Each serving provides
123 calories, 7 g protein, <1 g fat
(<1 g saturated fat), 24 g carbohydrate
(22 g sugars), 1 g fiber, 76 mg sodium

You can use any fresh or frozen fruit that purées easily in a blender, such as pears,
melon, pitted cherries, papaya, kiwi fruit or passion fruit. Ready-to-eat fruit can also
be found refrigerated in containers at the supermarket. Canned fruit is also fine—
it keeps well in the pantry. Choose canned fruit in natural juice, not syrup.

buttermilk & *pear smoothie*

SERVES 2   PREPARATION 10 MINUTES
COOKING NONE

1 ripe banana
2 ripe pears
1 vanilla bean or $^1/_2$ teaspoon
  (2 ml) vanilla extract
1 tablespoon (15 ml) orange juice
1 tablespoon (15 ml) pear juice
  concentrate
1 cup (250 ml) buttermilk
$^1/_4$ teaspoon (1 ml) ground cinnamon
$^2/_3$ cup (150 ml) mineral water

1 Peel and dice the banana. Peel and
quarter the pears and remove the
cores. Set aside two pear quarters
for garnish and dice the remainder.
2 If using a vanilla bean, halve the
bean lengthwise and scrape out the
seeds with the tip of a sharp knife.
3 Combine the banana and pears,
vanilla seeds or extract, orange
juice, pear juice concentrate,
buttermilk and half of the
cinnamon in a blender and
blend until smooth.
4 Stir the mineral water into the
mixture to thin it a little, then pour
the smoothie into two glasses.
Garnish each with a pear quarter,
sprinkle with the remaining
cinnamon and serve.

Each serving provides
237 calories, 6 g protein, 2 g fat
(1 g saturated fat), 49 g carbohydrate
(41 g sugars), 5 g fiber, 62 mg sodium

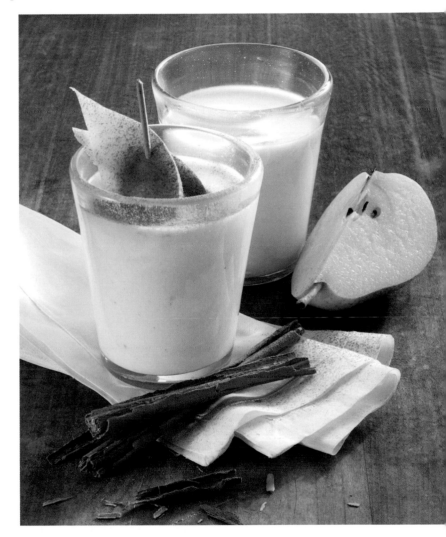

BUTTERMILK contains probiotics and
therefore supports good digestion.
It is also an excellent source of protein,
vitamin B_{12} for cell growth, potassium
for a healthy heart, and lecithin for
healthy nerve and brain function.

SERVES
2

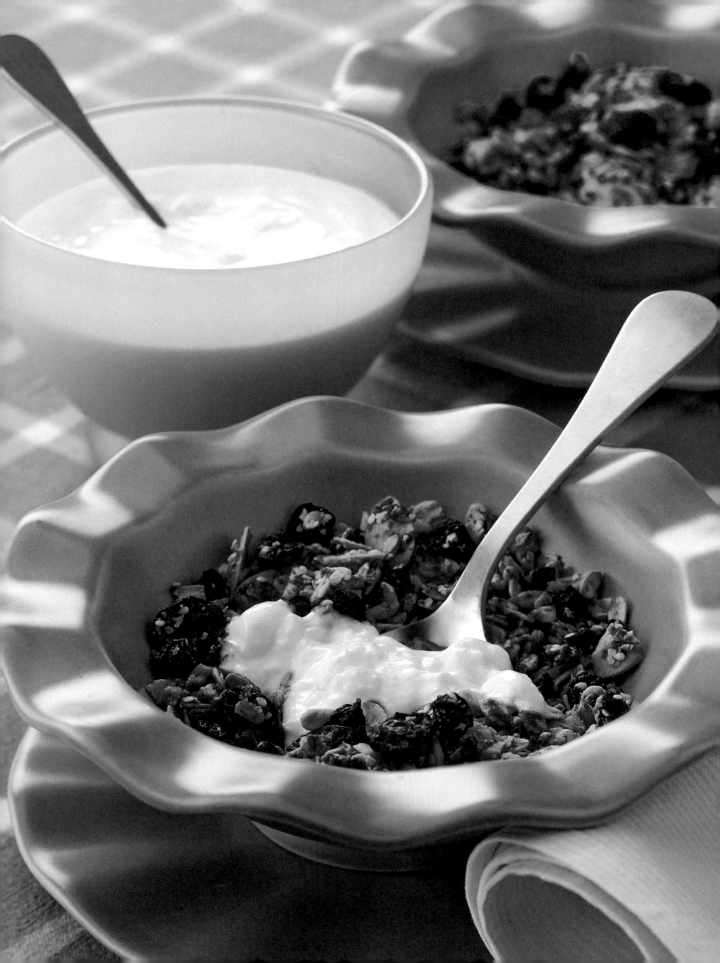

blueberry & *cranberry crunch*

Adding maple syrup and orange juice to a mix of grains, nuts and berries helps to keep this recipe lower in fat than most ready-made "crunchy" cereals. This delicious toasted muesli has a low GI, so make up a big batch that will last you for a week or two.

SERVES 8   PREPARATION 15 MINUTES   COOKING 30–40 MINUTES

2¼ cups (225 g) rolled oats

½ cup (50 g) wheat germ

⅔ cup (50 g) millet flakes

1 tablespoon (15 ml) sesame seeds

2 tablespoons (30 ml) sunflower seeds

2 tablespoons (30 ml) slivered almonds

½ cup (50 g) dried blueberries

½ cup (50 g) dried cranberries

1 tablespoon (15 ml) soft brown sugar

2 tablespoons (30 ml) pure maple syrup

2 tablespoons (30 ml) canola oil

2 tablespoons (30 ml) orange juice

1 Preheat the oven to 325°F (160°F). In a large bowl, combine the oats, wheat germ, millet flakes, sesame and sunflower seeds, almonds, dried berries and sugar. Stir until all the ingredients are thoroughly mixed.

2 Put the maple syrup, oil and orange juice in a small pitcher and whisk together. Pour this mixture slowly into the dry ingredients, stirring to be sure that the liquid is evenly distributed and coats everything lightly.

3 Spread the mixture out evenly on a nonstick baking pan. Bake for 30–40 minutes, or until slightly crisp and lightly browned. Stir the mixture every 10 minutes so it browns evenly.

4 Remove from the oven and let cool. Store in an airtight container for up to two weeks. Serve with low-fat plain yogurt, low-fat milk or fruit juice.

Each serving provides
282 calories, 6 g protein, 11 g fat (2 g saturated fat), 39 g carbohydrate (14 g sugars), 6 g fiber, 7 mg sodium

THIS BREAKFAST supplies plenty of fiber, B vitamins and essential fatty acids. Wheat germ is especially rich in B vitamins and vitamin E.

millet with stewed *dried fruit*

This breakfast will stop any mid-morning energy slumps: Dietary fiber and slower-releasing carbohydrates from the dried fruit, plus iron from the millet, provide you with sustained energy. Millet has a moderate GI. Combining it with dried fruit produces a lower GI meal.

SERVES
2

SERVES 2   PREPARATION 40 MINUTES, PLUS OVERNIGHT SOAKING   COOKING 35 MINUTES

4 dried apricots
4 pitted dried prunes
1 cup (120 g) millet
$\frac{1}{2}$ teaspoon (2 ml) ground cardamom
1 teaspoon (5 ml) vanilla sugar

1 Finely dice the dried fruit. Transfer to a bowl, cover with 1 cup (250 ml) of water and let soak overnight.

2 Rinse the millet in a sieve, then place in a small saucepan with 1¼ cups (300 ml) of water and briefly bring to a boil. Reduce the heat to very low, cover the pan and let the grains swell for about 30 minutes (or turn the heat off and let the pan sit on the stove).

3 Meanwhile, transfer the dried fruit and the soaking water to a saucepan, add the cardamom, then cover and simmer gently over medium heat for about 10 minutes. Remove from the heat and set aside to cool a little.

4 Fold the apricot and prune mixture into the millet. Divide the millet and fruit between two bowls, sprinkle with vanilla sugar and serve warm.

Each serving provides
275 calories, 8 g protein, 3 g fat (<1 g saturated fat), 54 g carbohydrate (14 g sugars), 8 g fiber, 11 mg sodium

MILLET contains all essential amino acids and is a rich source of silicic acid, which supports the body's own production of collagen and therefore plays an important role in maintaining healthy hair, skin, nails, teeth and eyes. This cereal provides an optimum combination of iron, magnesium, B vitamins and slower-releasing carbohydrates.

DRIED FRUIT is often treated with sulfur as a preservative to ensure that the fruit retains its color. If you are sensitive to sulfur dioxide, use unsulfured dried fruit.

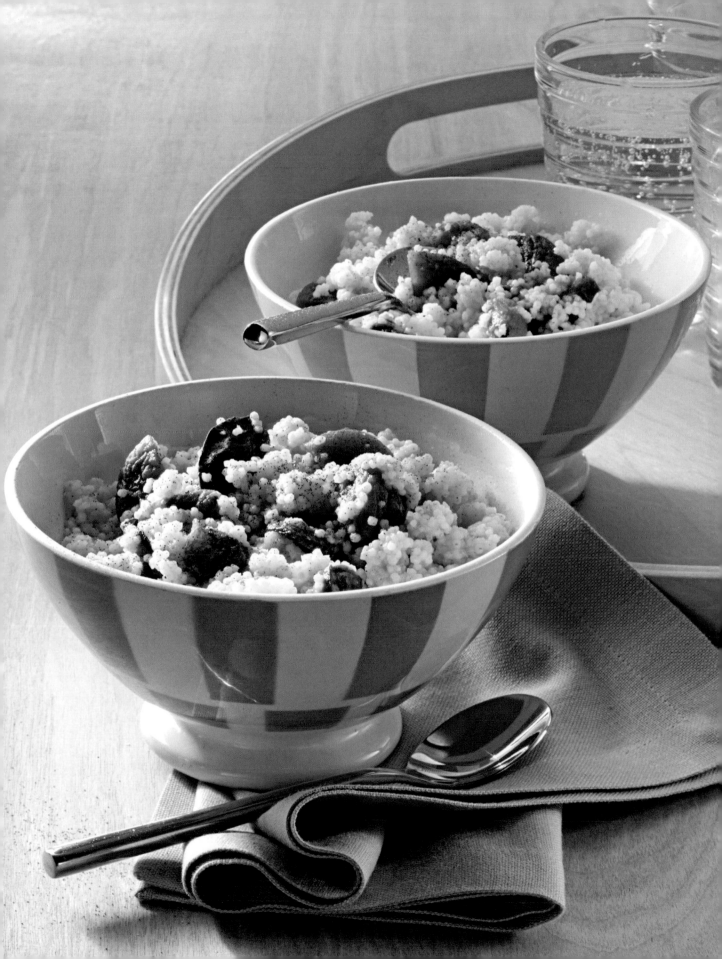

rhubarb & *strawberry compote*

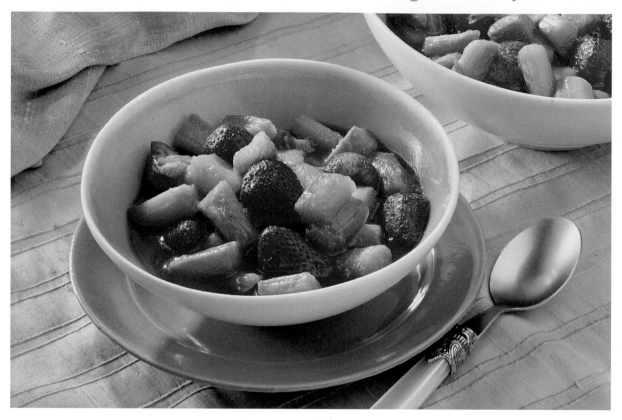

SERVES 4   PREPARATION 15 MINUTES
COOKING 15 MINUTES

1¼ pounds (625 g) rhubarb
¼ cup (50 g) superfine sugar
½ cup (125 ml) fresh orange juice
1⅔ cups (250 g) strawberries

1 Trim and rinse the rhubarb, and cut into 1 inch (2.5 cm) lengths. Put the rhubarb in a large saucepan with the sugar and orange juice. Cover and bring to a boil, reduce the heat and simmer gently, uncovered, for 5–6 minutes, stirring occasionally.

2 Meanwhile, hull the strawberries, and halve or quarter any large ones. Add to the pan and cook gently for another 4–5 minutes, or until slightly softened. They should maintain their shape and still have some bite.

3 Taste the fruit and add a little more sugar if necessary. Divide the compote among four bowls and serve while still warm. Serve topped with low-fat yogurt if you like.

Each serving provides
113 calories, 4 g protein, 0 g fat (0 g saturated fat),
20 g carbohydrate (20 g sugars), 5 g fiber, 25 mg sodium

fruity *muesli*

SERVES 4   PREPARATION 15 MINUTES,
PLUS OVERNIGHT SOAKING   COOKING NONE

1 cup (115 g) rolled oats
1 cup (115 g) raisins
1 cup (250 ml) low-fat milk
1 red or green apple
2 teaspoons (10 ml) lemon juice
$1/4$ cup (30 g) roughly
   chopped hazelnuts
2 tablespoons (30 ml) pumpkin seeds
1 tablespoon (15 ml) sesame seeds
$2/3$ cup (100 g) strawberries,
   hulled and chopped
4 tablespoons (60 ml) low-fat
   plain yogurt
4 teaspoons (20 ml) honey

1 Place the oats and raisins in a large
bowl and add the milk. Stir
to combine well, cover the bowl
and place in the refrigerator.
Let soak overnight.

2 The next day, just before eating,
grate the apple into a bowl. Toss
the apple with the lemon juice to
prevent the apple from browning.

3 Stir the hazelnuts, pumpkin seeds
and sesame seeds into the oat
mixture, then stir in the grated
apple and the strawberries.

4 Divide the muesli among four
serving bowls, and top each with
a spoonful of yogurt and honey.

Each serving provides
381 calories, 12 g protein, 12 g fat
(2 g saturated fat), 57 g carbohydrate
(38 g sugars), 7 g fiber, 70 mg sodium

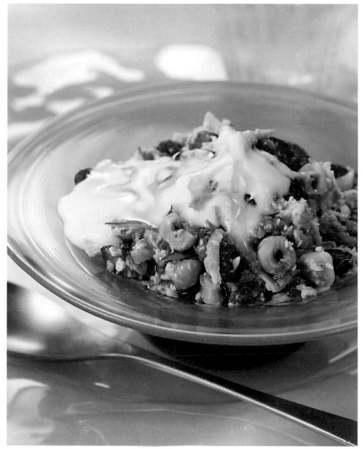

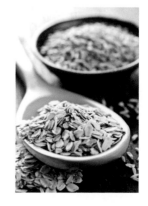

Superfood
OATS have a low GI and
produce a more gradual rise
in blood glucose levels. This
breakfast should keep you
satisfied until lunchtime.

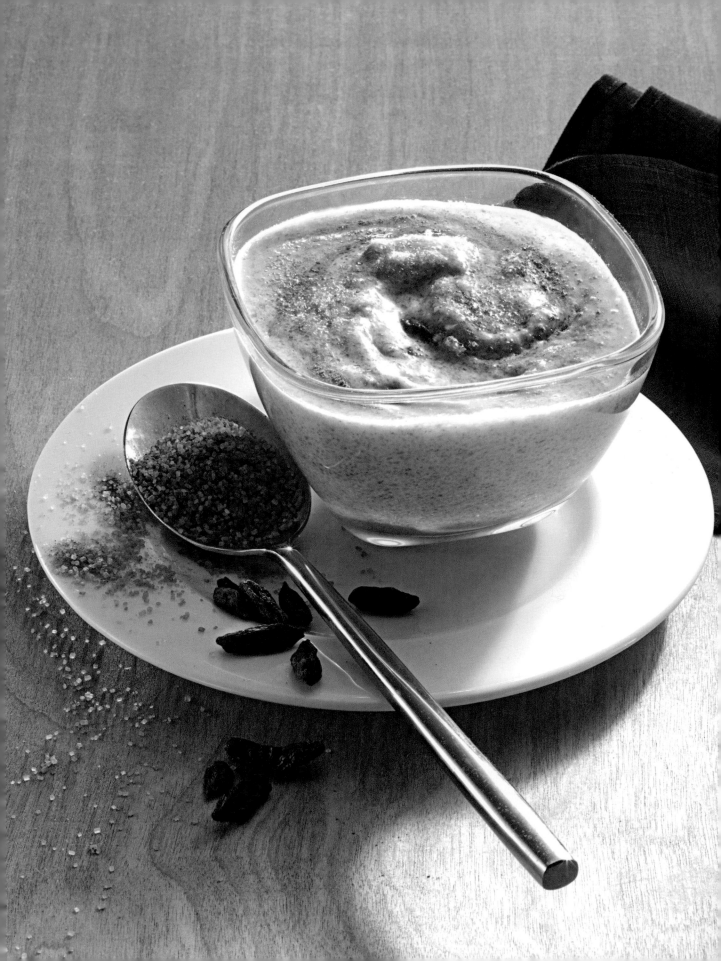

warm semolina cereal with *goji berries*

SERVES 2

Semolina is a processed form of durum (hard) wheat and is commonly used in puddings and cooked cereals or mixed with egg to make pasta. It's digested slowly and has a low glycemic index. Look for spelt semolina: It has a lovely nutty flavor.

SERVES 2   PREPARATION 10 MINUTES   COOKING 10 MINUTES

$1^2/_3$ cups (400 ml) almond, soy
  or rice milk
4 tablespoons (60 ml) semolina (use
  spelt semolina, if available)
2 tablespoons (30 ml) dried
  goji berries
2 tablespoons (30 ml)
  slivered almonds
2 teaspoons (10 ml) honey
1 teaspoon (5 ml) ground cinnamon
1 teaspoon (5 ml) raw sugar

1 Pour the milk into a saucepan and bring just to a boil over low heat, and slowly whisk in the semolina, stirring constantly. Add the goji berries, almonds, honey and half of the cinnamon.
2 Bring the cereal to a boil and cook for another 2–3 minutes, or until thickened, stirring continuously. Remove the pan from the heat and let rest for a few minutes.
3 Combine the remaining cinnamon with the sugar. Divide the semolina between two bowls. Sprinkle with the cinnamon sugar and serve warm.

ANOTHER IDEA
+ *If you prefer, this cereal can be prepared with low-fat milk or water. Simply add the semolina to the milk or water in a slow, steady stream and cook as in step 1.*

Each serving provides
265 calories, 7 g protein, 8 g fat (1 g saturated fat),
41 g carbohydrate (21 g sugars), 4 g fiber, 155 mg sodium

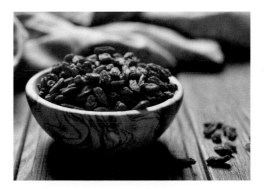

Superfood
GOJI BERRIES contain many health-promoting compounds: 19 amino acids, 21 trace elements, more vitamin C than oranges, more protein than whole-grain wheat, plus vitamin E, B vitamins, carotenoids, essential fatty acids and a whole range of other nutrients to strengthen the heart and blood vessels, brain and muscles. All dried fruits are high in natural sugars, so limit yourself to 1–2 tablespoons (15–30 ml) per day.

raisin & nut-studded
amaranth cereal

Amaranth is a very nutritious high-protein grain and is used in soups, stews and sweet dishes, or can be ground into flour for use in pastas and baked goods. In this homey breakfast dish, the amaranth retains its crunchy texture, and its nutty flavor is further emphasized by the addition of pine nuts.

SERVES 6   PREPARATION 15 MINUTES   COOKING 40 MINUTES

3 cups (750 ml) low-fat milk

1 cup (250 g) whole-grain amaranth

$1/4$ cup (50 g) soft brown sugar
  or maple sugar

2 teaspoons (10 ml) finely grated
  orange zest, plus extra to garnish

2 teaspoons (10 ml) finely grated
  lemon zest, plus extra to garnish

$1/4$ teaspoon (1 ml) ground
  cardamom

2 tablespoons (30 ml) pine nuts

$1/3$ cup (40 g) raisins, plus extra
  to garnish

$1/2$ teaspoon (2 ml) vanilla extract

1 Combine the milk, amaranth, sugar, orange zest, lemon zest and cardamom in a large saucepan over medium heat and bring to a boil. Reduce the heat to low, cover and simmer for 35 minutes, stirring occasionally, or until the amaranth is tender.

2 Remove from the heat and stir in the pine nuts, raisins and vanilla. Spoon the cereal into serving bowls or glasses and garnish with the extra zest and the raisins. Serve at room temperature, or refrigerate if you prefer and serve chilled.

Each serving provides
309 calories, 13 g protein, 6 g fat (1 g saturated fat),
50 g carbohydrate (22 g sugars), 7 g fiber, 90 mg sodium

AMARANTH is a very good source of fiber. Cultivated since ancient times, amaranth is also rich in magnesium, iron and the amino acid lysine (which is rare in plant sources). Most major supermarkets now stock amaranth and you'll also find it in health food stores.

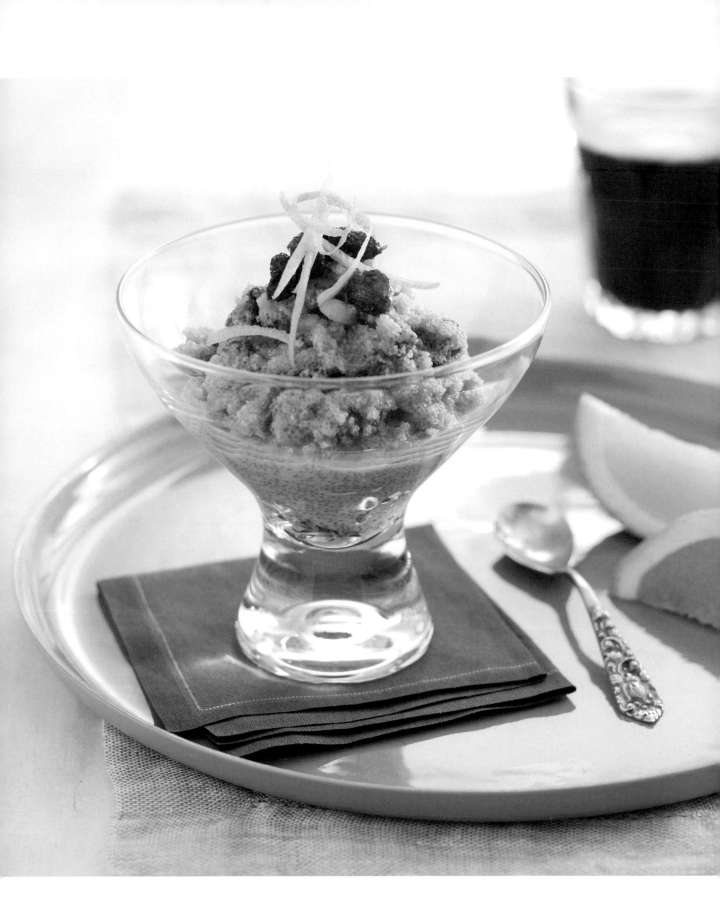

breakfast bread *pudding*

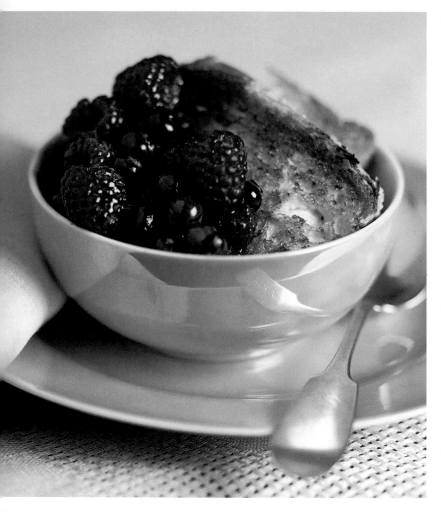

SERVES 6   PREPARATION 10 MINUTES, PLUS
20 MINUTES STANDING   COOKING 40 MINUTES

¹/₄ cup (55 g) sugar
2 large eggs
3 large egg whites
2 cups (500 ml) low-fat milk
1 teaspoon (5 ml) vanilla extract
olive oil spray, for greasing
8 slices whole-grain bread, toasted
2 cups (310 g) blueberries
2 cups (250 g) raspberries

1 Put 2 tablespoons (30 ml) sugar in
  a bowl. Add the eggs, egg whites,
  milk and vanilla and whisk together
  until combined.
2 Spray a 8-inch (20-cm) square baking
  dish with olive oil spray. Place four
  slices of toast in the bottom of the
  baking dish, then pour half the
  egg mixture evenly over the top.
  Repeat with the remaining toast
  and egg mixture. Allow to stand for
  20 minutes.
3 Meanwhile, preheat the oven to 350°F
  (180°C). Place the baking dish in a
  large roasting pan. Put the roasting
  pan on an oven rack and pour in
  enough hot water to come halfway up
  the outside of the baking dish. Bake
  for 40 minutes, or until the pudding is
  set and the top is golden and puffed.
  Remove from oven and cool slightly.
4 In a bowl, toss the berries with
  the remaining sugar. Serve the
  bread pudding warm, topped with
  the berries.

Each serving provides
245 calories, 13 g protein, 4 g fat
(1 g saturated fat), 38 g carbohydrate
(24 g sugars), 6 g fiber, 299 mg sodium

BERRIES are nutritionally very powerful,
with a remarkable fiber and antioxidant
content for their size. Use frozen berries
when fresh are out of season.

buttermilk pancakes

SERVES 4 (MAKES 12) PREPARATION
20 MINUTES COOKING 15 MINUTES

1 1/2 cups (220 g) whole-wheat
   self-rising flour
2 tablespoons (30 ml) superfine sugar
2 large eggs, separated
1 1/4 cups (300 ml) reduced-fat
   buttermilk
1 large banana, thinly sliced
2 teaspoons (10 ml) sunflower oil

To serve (optional)
1/3 cup (90 ml) Greek-style yogurt
   mixed with 1/4 teaspoon (1 ml)
   ground cinnamon
1 1/2 tablespoons (22 ml) honey

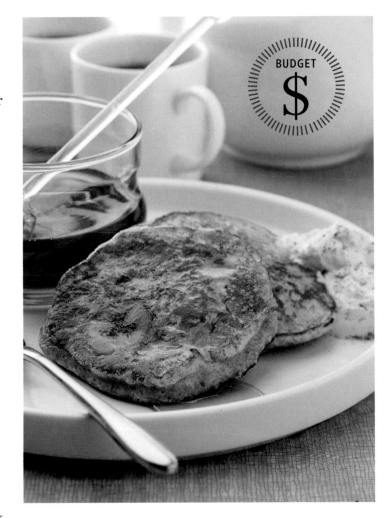

1 Sift the flour into a large bowl,
   and add the bran that's left in the
   sieve. Stir in the sugar. Mix the
   egg yolks with the buttermilk and
   1 tablespoon (15 ml) cold water.
   Gradually beat the buttermilk
   mixture into the flour to make a
   very thick batter.
2 Whisk the egg whites in a separate
   bowl until light and fluffy. Fold into
   the batter, then fold in the banana.
3 Heat a large heavy-bottom, nonstick
   frying pan over medium heat, and
   lightly grease with a little of the oil.
   Spoon large, heaping spoonfuls of
   the batter into the hot pan, spacing
   them well apart. You'll probably be
   able to cook three or four at a time,
   depending on the size of the pan.
4 Cook the pancakes until golden and
   firm on the underside and bubbles
   appear on the surface. Flip the pancakes with a spatula
   and cook for another 1–2 minutes. Remove and keep
   warm while cooking the rest of the pancakes, lightly
   greasing the pan with more oil between each batch.
5 Serve the pancakes warm, topped with a dollop of
   spiced yogurt and drizzled with honey, if you like.

Each serving (3 pancakes) provides
333 calories, 14 g protein, 8 g fat (2 g saturated fat),
51 g carbohydrate (17 g sugars), 7 g fiber, 445 mg sodium

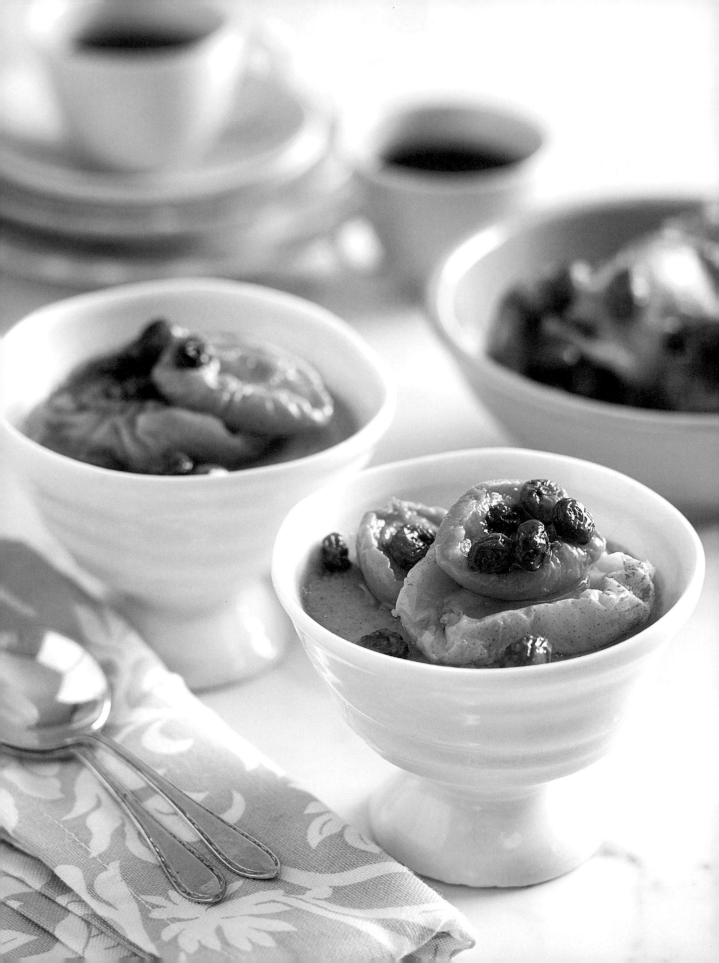

cinnamon &
banana yogurt whip

Here's a bowl of breakfast goodness that's low in fat and high in fiber. Using freshly ground cinnamon instead of the ready-ground version will give you a greater depth of flavor and aroma. Cinnamon sticks can be grated using a microplane grater, or ground in a mortar and pestle, a blender or a spice grinder.

SERVES 4 PREPARATION 10 MINUTES,
PLUS OVERNIGHT SOAKING AND CHILLING
COOKING NONE

4 dried apricot halves
4 dried peach halves
4 dried pear halves
1/4 cup (30 g) raisins
2 teaspoons (10 ml) ground cinnamon or a 1 1/2 inch (4 cm) cinnamon stick
2 tablespoons (30 ml) wheat germ
2 large bananas
2 tablespoons (30 ml) honey
1 cup (250 ml) low-fat plain yogurt
1 teaspoon (5 ml) powdered gelatin

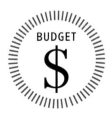
BUDGET
$

1 Place the dried apricots, peaches, pears and raisins in a small bowl and pour in enough cold water to cover the fruit. Cover the bowl and let the fruit soak in the refrigerator overnight.

2 Put the cinnamon and wheat germ in a food processor or blender and process briefly until finely ground. Add the bananas and honey and process until smooth. Stir the yogurt into the banana mixture to combine well.

3 Pour 3 tablespoons (45 ml) water into a large heatproof bowl and sprinkle with the gelatin. Warm the gelatin in the microwave, or over a saucepan of boiling water, until it dissolves completely. Slowly pour the banana yogurt mixture into the gelatin, stirring rapidly.

4 Divide the yogurt mixture among four small bowls or glasses. Put in the refrigerator to set overnight.

5 To serve, put the soaked fruit into a sieve to drain off the liquid, then divide the fruit among the bowls.

ANOTHER IDEA

+ *The gelatin used in the yogurt whips sets overnight, at the same time that the dried fruit are soaking. For a quicker version that you can serve immediately after making, omit the gelatin and dried fruit and serve the yogurt whips topped with slices of fresh fruit.*

Each serving provides
235 calories, 7 g protein, 1 g fat (<1 g saturated fat),
52 g carbohydrate (45 g sugars), 6 g fiber, 48 mg sodium

fruit & nut oatmeal

There is nothing more comforting and nutritious than a bowl of warm oatmeal to start the day, not only in winter but throughout the year, changing the fruit topping according to what's in season. The hazelnuts and almond meal boost the protein content, helping to make you feel full for longer. Grapes add natural sweetness.

SERVES 1 PREPARATION 5 MINUTES COOKING 10 MINUTES

$1/2$ cup (50 g) rolled oats
$1/2$ cup (125 ml) low-fat milk
1 tablespoon (15 ml) almond meal
2 teaspoons (10 ml) wheat germ
1 tablespoon (15 ml) chopped
   hazelnuts, toasted
$1/2$ cup (90 g) black grapes, halved

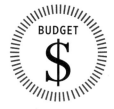

BUDGET $

1 Put the oats, milk and $1/2$ cup (125 ml) water in a small saucepan over medium heat. Bring to a boil, reduce the heat to low and simmer for about 5 minutes, stirring regularly, until the oats have thickened and are cooked through.
2 Stir in the almond meal, and pour the oatmeal into a serving bowl. Sprinkle the wheat germ on top, followed by the hazelnuts and grapes.

OTHER IDEAS

+ *Swap the grapes with berries, such as blackberries, raspberries or blueberries.*
+ *If you don't have any fresh fruit, canned fruit (preferably canned in fruit juice or water with no added sugar) makes a handy year-round substitute.*
+ *Add more crunch by finely chopping up a sweet red or green apple and adding it instead of the grapes.*

Each serving provides
425 calories, 16 g protein, 16 g fat (3 g saturated fat), 53 g carbohydrate (23 g sugars), 8 g fiber, 84 mg sodium

HAZELNUTS contain "good" fats, but you still need to limit your portions. If you're eating them as a snack, stick to a small handful (no more than 20) at a time.

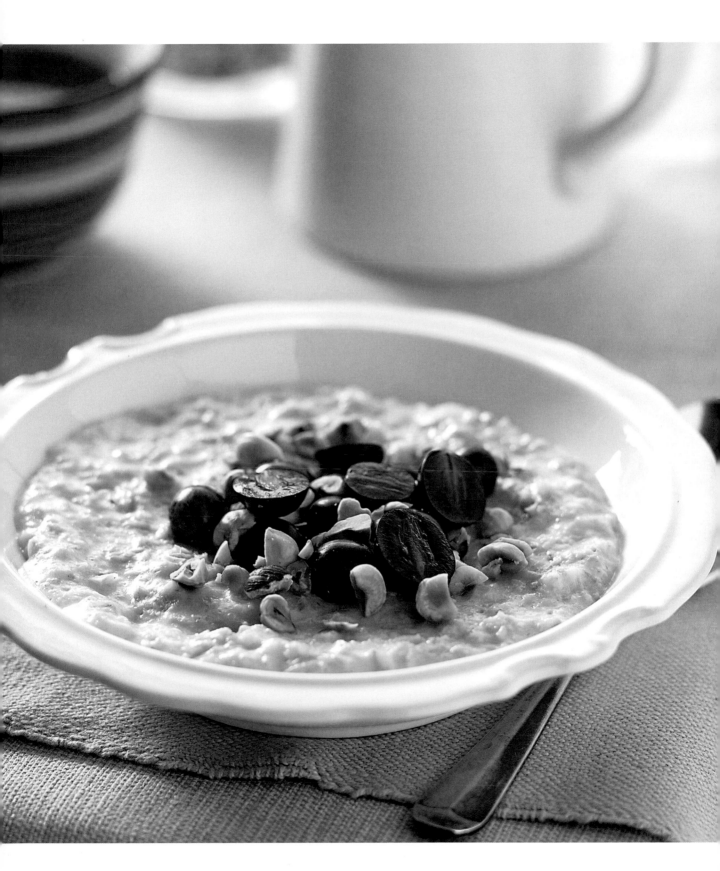

SERVES
2

oatmeal with *summer fruit*

Oatmeal is a sustaining breakfast with a low glycemic index. Make sure you use traditional slow-cooking oats and not the instant, quick-cook type, as these don't have the same health benefits as coarser traditional oats.

SERVES 2   PREPARATION 5 MINUTES   COOKING 10 MINUTES

$^1/_2$ cup (50 g) rolled oats
$^1/_3$ cup (90 ml) low-fat plain yogurt
$^2/_3$ cup (85 g) fresh raspberries
$^1/_2$ cup (80 g) fresh blueberries
2 teaspoons (10 ml) soft brown sugar

1 Put the oats and 2 cups (500 ml) water in a small saucepan. Bring to a boil, reduce the heat to low and simmer for about 5 minutes, stirring regularly, until the oats have thickened and are cooked through.

2 Divide the oatmeal between two bowls and top each with 2 tablespoons (30 ml) of yogurt. Scatter the berries on top, then sprinkle each serving with a teaspoon (5 ml) of brown sugar.

OTHER IDEAS

+ *Use other fresh fruit if you prefer, such as sliced mangoes, apricots, peaches, or stewed apples or pears in winter.*
+ *Instead of using brown sugar, sweeten the oatmeal with a drizzle of pure maple syrup or honey.*

Each serving provides
165 calories, 6 g protein, 2 g fat (1 g saturated fat),
27 g carbohydrate (12 g sugars), 5 g fiber, 35 mg sodium

OATS contain a special type of soluble fiber called beta-glucan, which helps to bind cholesterol and remove it from the body. Beta-glucan works best when eaten as part of the whole oat grain, because then it can work together with other beneficial substances that oats provide. Both oats and berries contain heart-protective antioxidants as well.

blueberry popovers

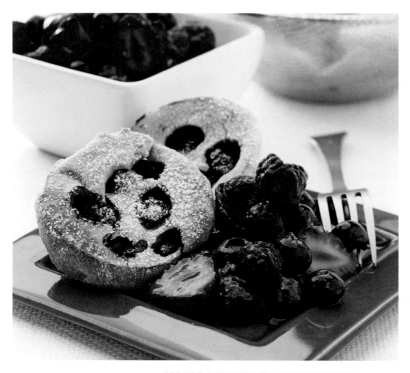

SERVES 4 (MAKES 8)   PREPARATION
20 MINUTES   COOKING 30 MINUTES

1 teaspoon (5 ml) butter, for greasing
3/4 cup (110 g) all-purpose flour
pinch of salt
1 teaspoon (5 ml) superfine sugar
2 eggs
1 cup (250 ml) low-fat milk
1/2 cup (80 g) blueberries
1 tablespoon (15 ml) confectioners'
   sugar, to serve

Mixed berry salad
1 1/4 cups (150 g) raspberries
2/3 cup (100 g) blueberries
1 1/3 cups (200 g) strawberries, halved
1 tablespoon (15 ml) confectioners'
   sugar, to taste

1 Preheat the oven to 425°F (220°C).
Use the butter to lightly grease eight
cups of a deep 12-hole muffin pan.
2 To make the popovers, sift the flour,
salt and superfine sugar into a
mixing bowl and make a well in the
center. Break the eggs into the well,
add the milk and beat with a fork.
3 Using a whisk, gradually work the
flour into the liquid to make a smooth
batter that has the consistency of
heavy cream. Pour into a pitcher.
4 Pour the batter into the prepared
pan, filling the cups two-thirds full.
With a spoon, drop a few blueberries
into the batter in each cup, dividing
them equally.
5 Bake for 25–30 minutes, or until the
popovers are golden brown, puffed
up and crisp around the edges.
6 Meanwhile, make the berry salad.
Purée 1/2 cup (125 g) of the
raspberries by pressing them
through a nylon sieve into a bowl.
Add the rest of the raspberries to the
bowl, together with the blueberries
and strawberries. Sift the
confectioners' sugar over the fruit
and fold gently to combine.
7 Unmold the popovers with a round-
bladed knife, then dust the tops with
the confectioners' sugar. Serve hot,
with the berry salad.

Each serving provides
244 calories, 11 g protein, 4 g fat
(2 g saturated fat), 40 g carbohydrate
(20 g sugars), 5 g fiber, 236 mg sodium

yogurt berry parfaits

SERVES 4   PREPARATION 15 MINUTES
COOKING NONE

2 cups (250 g) fresh or frozen mixed
   berries, such as strawberries,
   raspberries and blackberries
1 tablespoon (15 ml) lemon juice
2 tablespoons (30 ml)
   superfine sugar
1 cup (125 g) reduced-fat muesli
$\frac{1}{2}$ cup (50 g) walnut halves,
   roughly chopped
1 pomegranate (optional)
$1^2/_3$ cups (400 ml) low-fat
   Greek-style yogurt

1 Chill four tall glasses in the fridge.
2 Combine the berries, lemon juice
   and sugar in a food processor or
   blender and process to make a
   smooth coulis.
3 Put the muesli and walnuts in a
   bowl and stir to combine well.
4 If using the pomegranate, fill a
   large bowl with water. Cut the top
   off the pomegranate, then cut into
   quarters. Hold the pomegranate
   under the water in the bowl (this
   prevents the juice squirting) and
   gently bend the skin back to open
   the membranes; pry out the seeds.
   The bitter white membranes will
   float to the top and the seeds will
   sink. Scoop out the membranes,
   then drain the seeds in a sieve.
5 Put a spoonful of the muesli
   mixture in the bottom of each

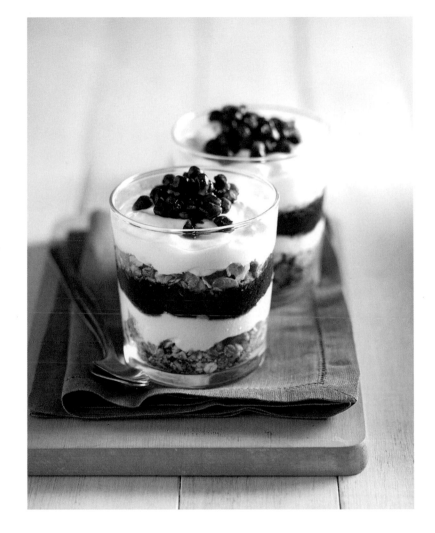

glass. Top with a spoonful of yogurt, then add a thick
layer of berry coulis. Repeat until each glass is filled.
Top with pomegranate seeds or a spoonful of coulis
to serve.

Each serving provides
375 calories, 13 g protein, 13 g fat (3 g saturated fat),
50 g carbohydrate (29 g sugars), 6 g fiber, 178 mg sodium

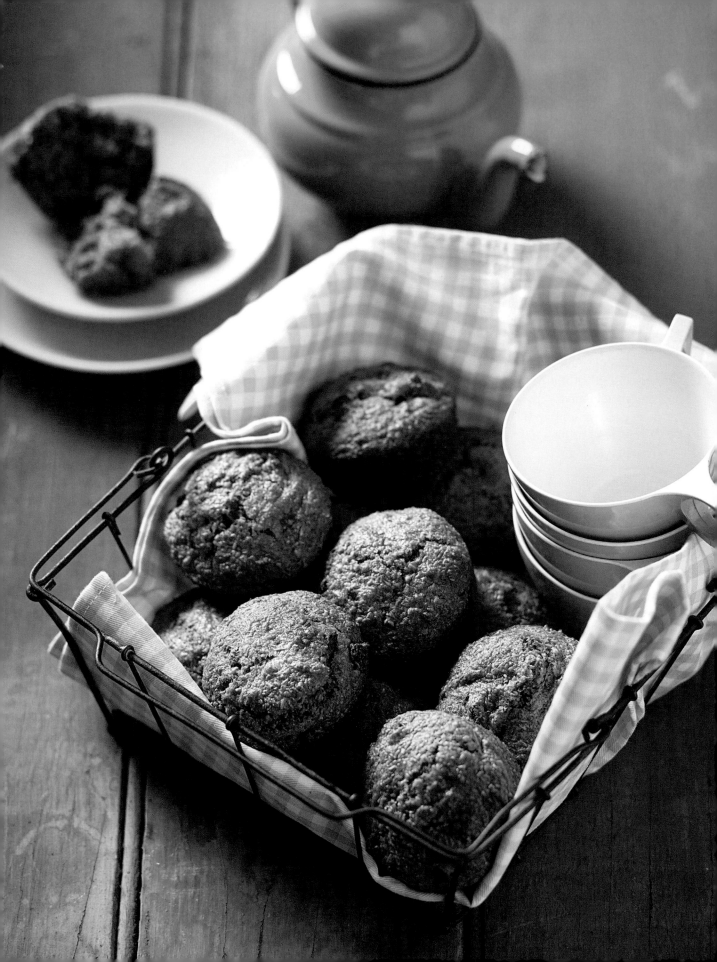

spicy bran & *goji berry muffins*

Goji berries are related to the chile family and resemble very small pale red chilies. Usually sold dried, goji berries have a sweet, tangy flavor and are very high in antioxidants, vitamins and minerals. With goji berries, walnuts for omega-3 oils and a blend of spices, these are the ultimate antioxidant high-fiber snack.

MAKES 12   PREPARATION 15 MINUTES, PLUS OVERNIGHT STANDING   COOKING 25 MINUTES

1 cup (150 g) self-rising flour
1 teaspoon (5 ml) ground
   mixed spice
1 teaspoon (5 ml) baking soda
$^1/_2$ cup (115 ml) firmly packed
   soft brown sugar
$1^2/_3$ cups (100 g) unprocessed
   wheat bran
$^1/_2$ cup (60 g) goji berries
   or currants
$^1/_2$ cup (60 g) chopped walnuts
1 egg
$1^1/_4$ cups (300 ml) buttermilk
$^1/_3$ cup (75 ml) canola oil
2 teaspoons (10 ml) canola oil,
   for greasing

1 Sift the flour, mixed spice and baking soda into a mixing bowl. Stir in the sugar, bran, goji berries and walnuts. Put the egg, buttermilk and oil in a separate bowl and whisk until combined.

2 Stir the egg mixture into the dry ingredients, but do not overmix; it should remain lumpy. Cover the bowl and leave in the refrigerator overnight.

3 Preheat the oven to 350°F (180°C). Grease a 12-hole standard muffin pan.

4 Spoon the batter into the prepared pan, filling the cups two-thirds full. Bake for 20–25 minutes, or until a skewer inserted in the center of a muffin comes out clean. Let the muffins cool in the pan for 5 minutes, then turn out onto a wire rack to finish cooling. Store in an airtight container for two days, or in the freezer for up to two months.

Each muffin provides
221 calories, 5 g protein, 12 g fat (1 g saturated fat), 25 g carbohydrate (12 g sugars), 3 g fiber, 161 mg sodium

WHEAT BRAN is a source of insoluble fiber, which helps to keep the digestive system and bowels healthy. Soluble fiber (found in oats, barley, legumes, pysllium) helps to manage cholesterol.

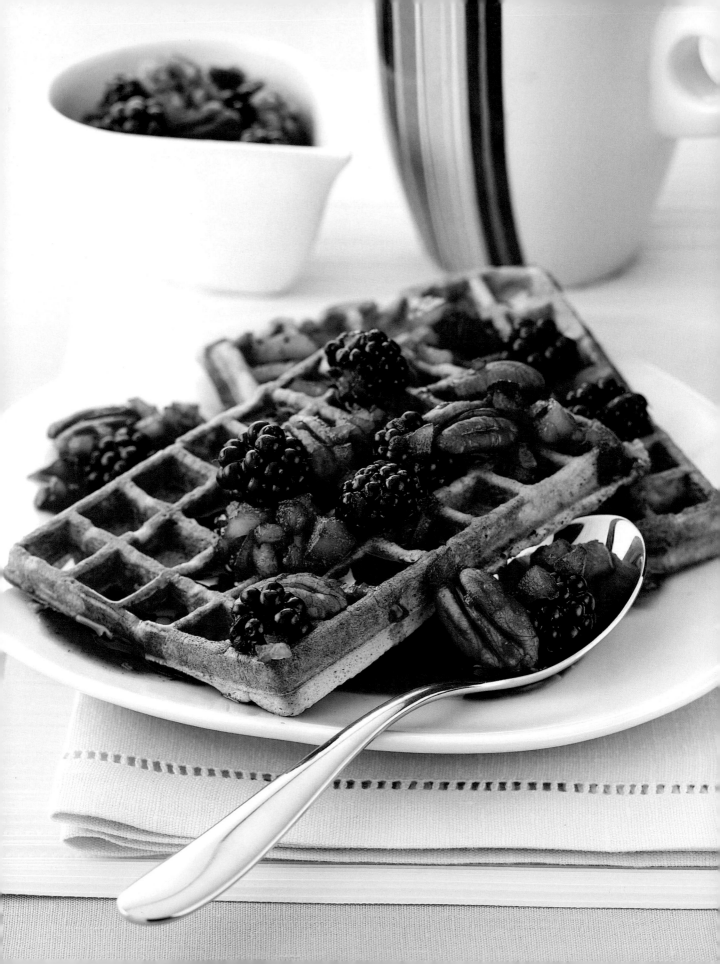

waffles with *blackberry sauce*

Crisp, crunchy waffles, so popular in France, Belgium and the U.S, too, are a lovely treat for breakfast or brunch. To make these you will need a waffle iron that can be used on the stovetop or an electric waffle maker.

SERVES 4 (MAKES ABOUT 8 WAFFLES)   PREPARATION 20 MINUTES   COOKING 15 MINUTES

1 teaspoon (5 ml) butter,
 for greasing
$^3/_4$ cup (110 g) all-purpose flour
$^1/_2$ teaspoon (2 ml) ground cinnamon
1 teaspoon (5 ml) baking powder
1 tablespoon (15 ml) superfine sugar
1 large egg, separated
1 cup (250 ml) low-fat milk
1 tablespoon (15 ml) butter, melted
$1^1/_2$ tablespoons (22 ml) finely
 chopped pecans

Blackberry sauce
1 large, ripe pear
$^1/_3$ cup (75 ml) pure maple syrup
$^1/_2$ cup (50 g) pecans
$^3/_4$ cup (100 g) blackberries

Each serving (2 waffles) provides
426 calories, 9 g protein, 19 g fat
(5 g saturated fat), 56 g carbohydrate
(32 g sugars), 5 g fiber, 158 mg sodium

1 To make the maple and blackberry sauce, cut the pear lengthwise into quarters and cut out the core, then cut the pear into small dice. Put the pear and maple syrup in a small heavy-bottom saucepan over low heat to warm through, then remove from the heat. Stir in the pecans and blackberries. Set aside.

2 Heat and lightly grease the waffle iron or electric waffle maker according to the manufacturer's instructions.

3 Meanwhile, to make the batter, sift the flour, cinnamon, baking powder and sugar into a bowl. Make a well in the center, then add the egg yolk and milk to the well. Gently whisk the egg yolk and milk together, and gradually whisk in the flour to make a thick, smooth batter. Whisk in the melted butter, and stir in the chopped pecans.

4 Whisk the egg white in a separate bowl until stiff peaks form. Pile the egg white on top of the batter and, using a large metal spoon, fold it in gently.

5 Spoon 3–4 tablespoons (45–60 ml) of batter into the center of the hot waffle iron or maker, then close the lid tightly. If using a waffle iron on the stovetop, cook for about 30 seconds, then turn the waffle iron over and cook for another 30 seconds. Open the waffle iron: The waffle should be golden brown on both sides and should come away easily from the iron. If using an electric waffle maker, follow the manufacturer's instructions (usually allow 2–3 minutes for each waffle). Keep warm while cooking the rest of the waffles.

6 Just before all the waffles are ready, gently warm the fruit sauce. Serve with the warm waffles.

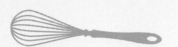

Make a batch of muffins for the week. They will keep for a couple of days, or you can wrap them individually in foil and freeze. Take out of the freezer and allow to thaw overnight, ready for a snack the next day.

wholesome *muffins*

Store-bought muffins have earned a bad reputation when it comes to healthy eating, but here is a recipe for a more virtuous kind using stone-ground flour, nuts and fruit. These muffins make the perfect mid-morning snack.

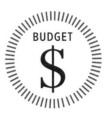

BUDGET
$

MAKES 12   PREPARATION 15 MINUTES   COOKING 20 MINUTES

1 teaspoon (5 ml) canola oil
2 eggs
1/2 cup (100 g) soft brown sugar
1 cup (250 g) diced apple
juice of 1/2 lemon
1 cup (250 ml) low-fat milk
3 tablespoons (45 ml) canola oil
1 teaspoon (5 ml) vanilla extract
1 cup (60 g) unprocessed
  wheat bran
1 cup (250 g) stone-ground
  whole-wheat flour
2 teaspoons (10 ml) baking powder
1 teaspoon (5 ml) baking soda
2 teaspoons (10 ml) ground
  cinnamon
1/2 teaspoon (2 ml) freshly
  grated nutmeg
pinch of salt
1/2 cup (85 g) blueberries
2 tablespoons (30 ml) chopped
  mixed nuts

1 Preheat the oven to 400°F (200°C). Lightly grease a deep 12-hole muffin pan with oil or line with paper cups.

2 Whisk the eggs and sugar together in a large mixing bowl until blended. In a small bowl, lightly crush the apples so that about half are still in shape, then stir into the egg mixture. Stir in the lemon juice. Combine the milk, oil and vanilla in another small bowl, then add to the egg and apple mixture. Add the bran and stir to combine well.

3 Combine the flour, baking powder, baking soda, spices and salt in a bowl, stirring well to combine the ingredients. Add this to the egg and bran mixture in the large bowl, stirring lightly until all the dry ingredients are incorporated. Fold in the blueberries.

4 Spoon the mixture into the muffin pan and sprinkle with the mixed nuts. Bake near the top of the oven for 15–20 minutes, or until a skewer inserted in the center of a muffin comes out clean. If not, give them another few minutes and check again. Don't let them overcook or they will be dry. Let the muffins cool in the pan for 5 minutes, then turn out onto a wire rack to finish cooling. Serve warm.

Each muffin provides
184 calories, 5 g protein, 8 g fat (1 g saturated fat),
24 g carbohydrate (12 g sugars), 5 g fiber, 159 mg sodium

STONE-GROUND FLOUR and wheat bran give these muffins a low GI. The apple and blueberries add natural sweetness and moisture.

APPLES AND BLUEBERRIES have a lower GI than the raisins often used in store-bought muffins.

poached eggs on *turkish toast*

This is an excellent breakfast with plenty of vitamin C from the tomatoes and scallions, and good-quality protein from the eggs. Poached eggs have much less fat than eggs that have been fried, scrambled or baked.

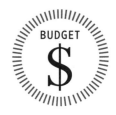

BUDGET
$

SERVES 4   PREPARATION 10 MINUTES   COOKING 5 MINUTES

6 ripe tomatoes, finely diced
3 scallions, thinly sliced
$\frac{1}{2}$ teaspoon (2 ml) ground sumac or paprika, plus extra to serve
freshly ground black pepper
4 eggs
Turkish bread

1 Combine the tomatoes and scallions in a bowl. Add the sumac and season to taste with pepper.
2 Fill a large shallow saucepan or deep frying pan with water and bring to a boil over a high heat. Reduce the heat to low, so the water is at a gentle simmer. Working with one egg at a time, crack the eggs into a cup and slide them into the simmering water. Poach for 3–4 minutes, or until the whites have set.
3 Meanwhile, split the bread horizontally, and cut it crosswise to make four square pieces. Toast each piece on both sides.
4 Remove the eggs from the pan with a slotted spoon and drain off the water. Place one egg on each piece of toast and spoon the tomato mixture on top. Sprinkle with extra sumac and serve immediately.

ANOTHER IDEA

+ *Substitute whole-grain pita bread for the Turkish bread, if preferred.*

Each serving provides
271 calories, 14 g protein, 7 g fat (2 g saturated fat), 38 g carbohydrate (6 g sugars), 5 g fiber, 444 mg sodium

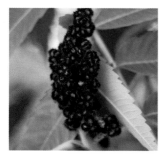

Food Fact
  SUMAC is a berry used in Middle Eastern cuisine. It has a slightly tangy citrus flavor and is sold in ground form in many large supermarkets and specialty food stores.

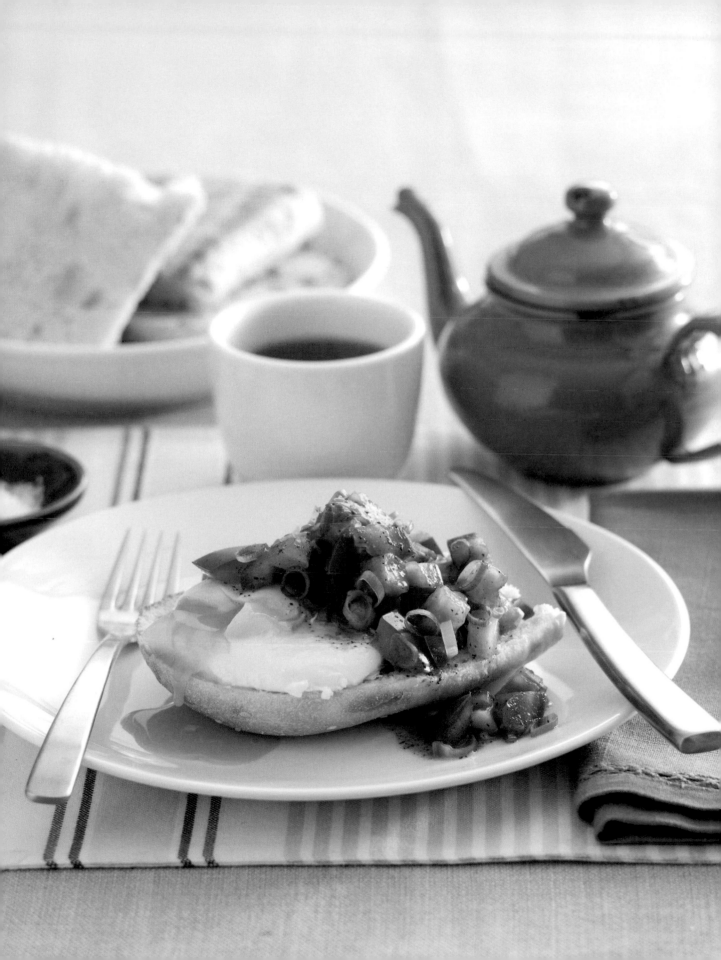

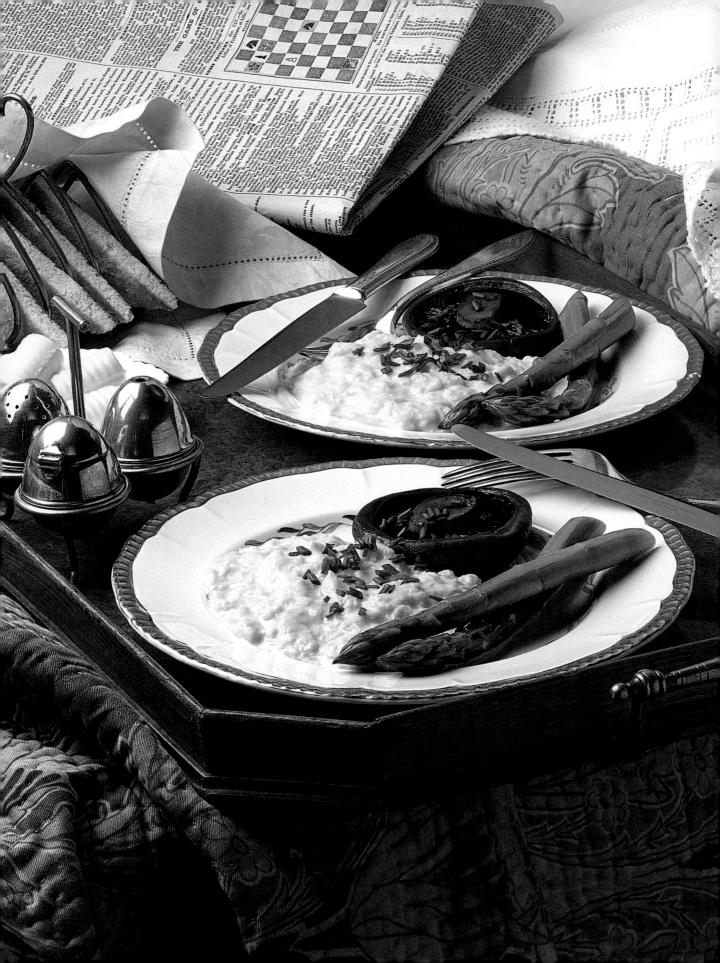

scrambled eggs with mushrooms & asparagus

Scrambled eggs don't have to be creamy, buttery affairs. Low-fat milk and heart-healthy olive oil, instead of cream and butter, help to keep the saturated fats low, making this an ideal breakfast choice. Mushrooms and asparagus provide fiber.

SERVES 4   PREPARATION 15 MINUTES   COOKING 15 MINUTES

1 tablespoon (15 ml) olive oil
4 large white or brown
   mushroom caps, wiped with a
   damp cloth
8 asparagus spears, trimmed
8 eggs
1/2 cup (125 ml) low-fat milk
freshly ground white pepper
8 slices whole-grain bread
1 tablespoon (15 ml) snipped
   fresh chives

1 Heat 2 teaspoons (10 ml) of the olive oil in a nonstick frying pan over low heat. Add the mushrooms, cover and cook for 10 minutes, or until the mushrooms are just softened. Steam the asparagus for 5–8 minutes, or until tender.

2 Meanwhile, beat the eggs with the milk in a bowl and season with a little white pepper. Heat the remaining oil in a heavy-bottom saucepan over a low heat. Add the egg mixture and stir gently until the eggs are just beginning to set. Remove from the heat and keep the eggs warm while you toast the bread. Cut the toast into triangles.

3 Spoon the scrambled eggs onto individual, warmed serving plates. Arrange the mushrooms and asparagus spears alongside the eggs. Sprinkle the eggs with chives and serve immediately with the triangles of toast.

Each serving provides
358 calories, 25 g protein, 17 g fat (4 g saturated fat),
27 g carbohydrate (5 g sugars), 7 g fiber, 451 mg sodium

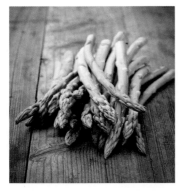

Superfood
   ASPARAGUS is an excellent source of dietary fiber and folate, and also contains a range of vitamins and minerals, including some B vitamins, vitamins A, C and K, manganese, copper and potassium.

french toast

This is a reduced-fat, high-protein version of French toast, made with evaporated milk, which has a creamy taste while being low in fat. The toast is served with mixed berries, which provide plenty of healthy antioxidants.

SERVES 4   PREPARATION 15 MINUTES   COOKING 10 MINUTES

2 eggs
1/2 cup (125 ml) light
   evaporated milk
2 teaspoons (10 ml) superfine sugar
1/2 teaspoon (2 ml) ground cinnamon
1 tablespoon (15 ml) olive oil spread
4 thick slices whole-grain
   sourdough bread
1 cup (250 g) fresh mixed berries
1/2 cup (125 ml) low-fat vanilla
   yogurt

1 Lightly whisk the eggs in a large bowl, add the milk and whisk until combined. Put the sugar and cinnamon in a small bowl and stir to combine.
2 Heat the olive oil spread in a large nonstick frying pan over medium heat.
3 Dip two slices of sourdough bread into the egg mixture, turning to coat well and allowing the excess to drip off. Place the bread in the hot pan and cook for 1–2 minutes on each side, or until golden brown. Transfer to a plate. Sprinkle with a little cinnamon sugar and cover to keep warm. Repeat with the remaining slices of bread.
4 Cut each piece of French toast in half and place on a plate. Top with some berries and a dollop of yogurt, and serve warm.

Each serving provides
262 calories, 11 g protein, 8 g fat (2 g saturated fat),
33 g carbohydrate (12 g sugars), 7 g fiber, 218 mg sodium

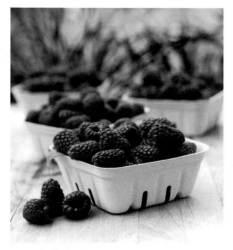

Superfood
   RASPBERRIES not only taste best when eaten as fresh as possible, but fresh raspberries are also richest in health-promoting vital nutrients. Raspberries are high in pectin, the soluble fiber that helps control blood cholesterol levels, and they contain ellagic acid, a phytochemical that is thought to neutralize carcinogens.

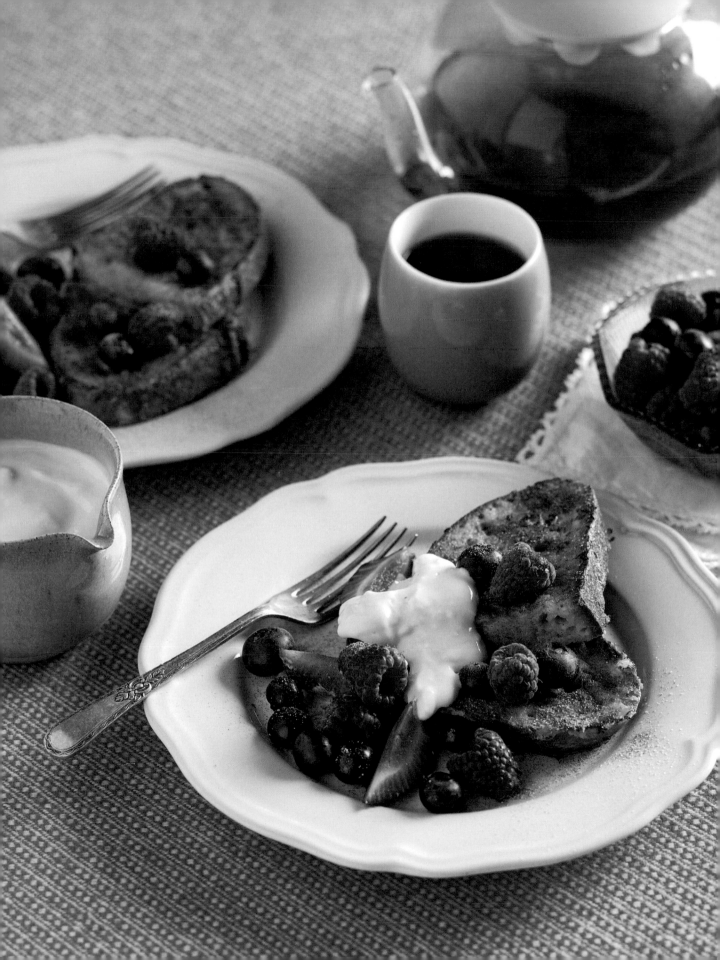

baked mushrooms *with ciabatta*

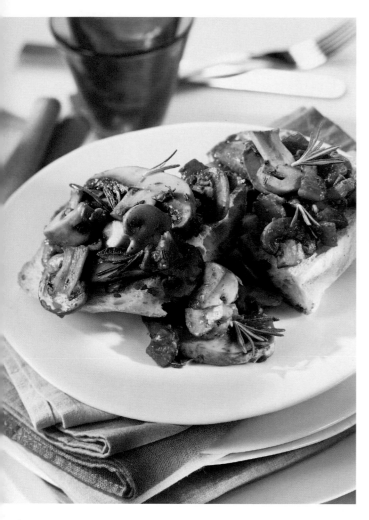

SERVES 4   PREPARATION 15 MINUTES
COOKING 20–25 MINUTES

3 cloves garlic, crushed

2 teaspoons (10 ml) lemon juice

$1^{1}/_{2}$ tablespoons (22 ml) olive oil

2 teaspoons (10 ml) balsamic vinegar

$^{1}/_{4}$ teaspoon (1 ml) freshly ground
black pepper, or to taste

2 cups (500 g) tomatoes, peeled, seeded
and chopped

2 pounds (1 kg) mixed button, cremini and
white mushrooms, sliced

2–4 sprigs of rosemary, leaves picked and
chopped, plus extra sprigs to garnish

1 teaspoon (5 ml) chopped fresh parsley or sage

4 large slices ciabatta bread

1 Preheat the oven to 400°F (200°C). Put the garlic,
lemon juice, oil, vinegar and pepper in a large
bowl and whisk to combine.

2 Add the tomatoes and mushrooms to the bowl
of dressing. Add the rosemary and parsley and
stir to combine well.

3 Spoon the tomato and mushroom mixture into a
baking dish and cover with foil. Make slits in the
top to release steam during cooking. Cook for
20–25 minutes, or until mushrooms are tender.

4 When they are nearly done, briefly heat the
bread in the oven. Place two slices of warmed
bread on each serving plate, cut side up, top with
the mushroom mixture and serve immediately,
garnished with the reserved rosemary.

Each serving provides

327 calories, 17 g protein, 10 g fat
(2 g saturated fat), 42 g carbohydrate
(4 g sugars), 11 g fiber, 396 mg sodium

MUSHROOMS are a useful source of fiber,
and contain energy-releasing B vitamins
and minerals, too. They are rich in
selenium, an important antioxidant that
may help to prevent heart disease and
cancer, as well as being high in folate for
healthy blood and circulation.

cottage cheese rolls
with kiwi fruit & orange

SERVES
2

SERVES 2 PREPARATION 10 MINUTES
COOKING NONE

$1/2$ cup (125 ml) low-fat
  cottage cheese
1 tablespoon (15 ml) orange juice
1 orange
1 golden kiwi fruit
2 sunflower seed bread rolls,
  halved
1 tablespoon (15 ml) honey, to drizzle
1–2 tablespoons (15–30 ml)
  sunflower seeds, toasted

1 Combine the cottage cheese with
the orange juice in a small bowl.
2 Peel the orange with a sharp knife,
leaving a little of the pith. Thinly
slice the fruit crosswise into circles.
Peel and slice the kiwi fruit.
3 Spread the bread roll halves with
the cottage cheese mixture.
4 Arrange orange and kiwis on the
rolls in overlapping slices. Drizzle
with honey and top with sunflower
seeds. Serve immediately.

ANOTHER IDEA
+ *Substitute chopped hazelnuts or
almonds for the sunflower seeds.
Use green kiwi fruit if golden is
not available.*

Each serving provides
400 calories, 25 g protein, 11 g fat
(3 g saturated fat), 47 g carbohydrate
(23 g sugars), 17 g fiber, 330 mg sodium

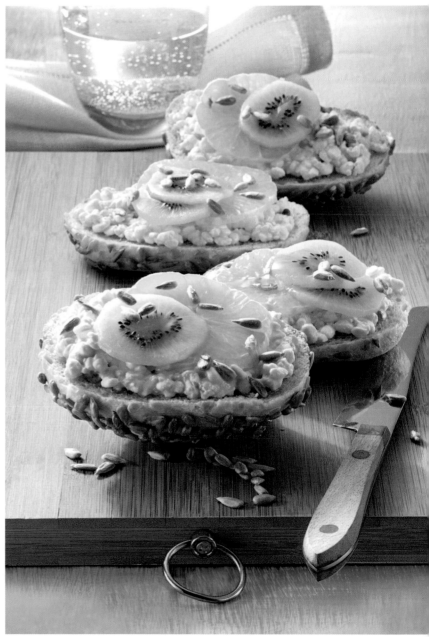

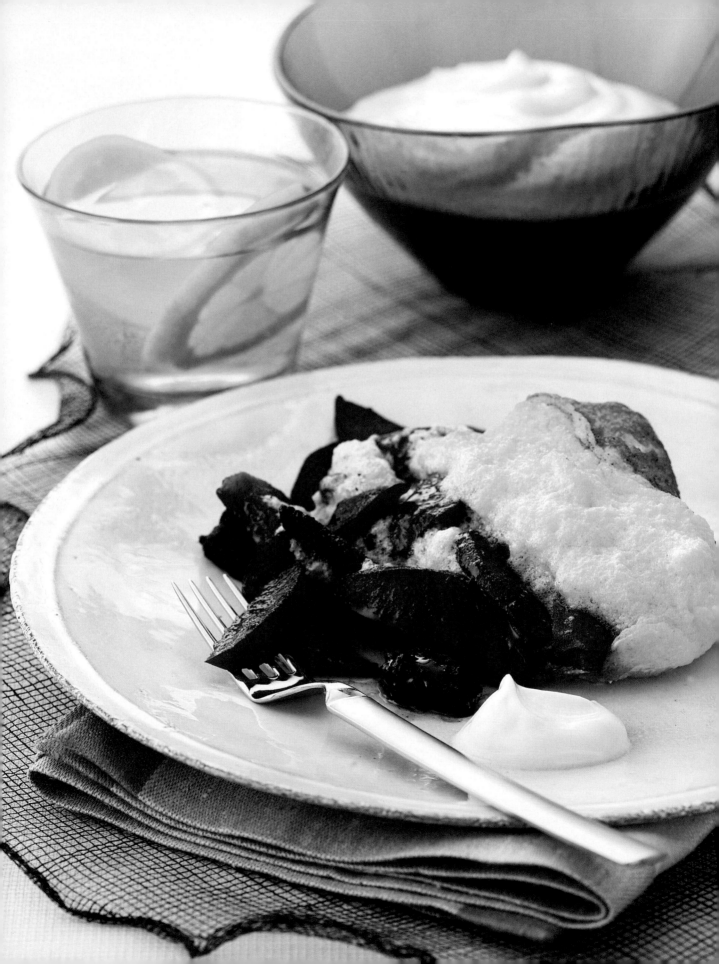

apple–berry *soufflé omelet*

This sweet omelet should be cooked just before serving so it stays puffed and warm. Serve it as a special weekend breakfast or brunch.

SERVES 2

SERVES 2   PREPARATION 15 MINUTES   COOKING 5 MINUTES

2 crisp sweet apples
$1/2$ cup (65 g) blackberries
$1/2$ teaspoon (2 ml) ground allspice
finely grated zest and juice of
   $1/2$ orange
2 eggs, separated
2 teaspoons (10 ml) superfine sugar
$1/2$ teaspoon (2 ml) vanilla extract
2 teaspoons (10 ml) canola oil
1 teaspoon (5 ml) raw sugar
2 tablespoons (30 ml) Greek-style
   yogurt

The use of eating apples instead of a cooking variety means that they need only light cooking and therefore not only retain their shape and texture, but also much of their nutritional value, too. They are naturally sweet, so require less added sugar.

1 Peel, core and thickly slice the apples. Put into a small saucepan and add the blackberries, allspice and orange juice. Cover the pan, place over low heat and cook for 2–3 minutes, shaking the pan occasionally, until the fruit juices release. Remove from heat and keep warm.

2 Put the egg yolks, sugar, orange zest and vanilla in a bowl and whisk together until smooth and thick.

3 In a separate, clean bowl, whisk the egg whites until they form soft peaks. Using a large spoon or spatula, fold the egg whites into the yolk mixture.

4 Preheat the broiler to medium. Meanwhile, heat the oil in a 8 inch (20 cm) nonstick frying pan with an ovenproof handle. Add the egg mixture, spreading it evenly, and cook over a low–medium heat for 2–3 minutes, or until set and golden on the bottom.

5 Place the pan under the broiler and cook for 1–2 minutes, or until the omelet is puffed and just set on top. Remove from the heat and turn the broiler to high.

6 Spoon the fruit mixture on top of the omelet and fold it over in half. Sprinkle with raw sugar and broil for about 30 seconds, or until the sugar caramelizes. Cut the omelet in half and serve immediately, topped with the yogurt.

Each serving provides
271 calories, 9 g protein, 12 g fat (3 g saturated fat),
33 g carbohydrate (32 g sugars), 5 g fiber, 83 mg sodium

oat *crepes*

Like the oatcakes of northern England, these fine-textured crepes are made with a blend of flour and ground rolled oats for extra fiber and a nutty flavor. In this recipe, nutrient-rich mushrooms are cooked in a low-fat white sauce for the filling.

SERVES 4 (MAKES 8)   PREPARATION 20 MINUTES, PLUS 15 MINUTES STANDING   COOKING 30 MINUTES

³/4 cup (110 g) whole-wheat flour
¹/3 cup (40 g) rolled oats
3 eggs
1 tablespoon (15 ml) olive oil, plus 1 tablespoon (15 ml) extra for frying
³/4 cup (175 ml) low-fat milk

Filling
2 tablespoons (30 ml) olive oil
1 small onion, finely chopped
1 clove garlic, crushed
1 cup (250 g) button mushrooms, thinly sliced
2 tablespoons (30 ml) all-purpose flour
1 cup (250 ml) low-fat milk
2 tablespoons (30 ml) finely snipped fresh chives

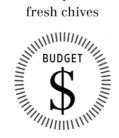

1 Put the whole-wheat flour and oats in a food processor or blender and process at high speed until finely ground. Place into a large bowl.

2 Put the eggs, 1 tablespoon (15 ml) oil and the milk in a pitcher and whisk until combined. Make a well in the center of the flour mixture and pour in the egg mixture. Whisk until smooth. Let the batter stand for 15 minutes.

3 Meanwhile, to make the filling, heat the oil in a large saucepan over a medium–high heat. Add the onion and cook, stirring, for 3–4 minutes, or until soft. Add the garlic and mushrooms and cook, stirring, for another 3–4 minutes, or until the mushrooms are tender.

4 Reduce the heat to medium. Sprinkle the flour evenly over the mushrooms and cook, stirring quickly, for 1 minute. Gradually stir in the milk until smooth. Cook, stirring, for 3–4 minutes, or until the mixture boils and thickens. Stir in the chives. Remove the pan from the heat and cover to keep warm.

5 Heat a little oil in a frying pan or crepe pan over medium heat. Spoon ¹/4 cup (50 ml) of batter into the pan and swirl to coat the base. Cook for 1 minute, turn and cook for another 1 minute, or until golden brown. Transfer to a plate and cover to keep warm. Repeat with the remaining batter to make eight crepes.

6 Divide the mushroom mixture among the crepes. Fold the crepes to enclose the filling and serve.

ANOTHER IDEA
+ *These oat crepes can be served spread with jam, or with fillings such as fresh berries and low-fat vanilla yogurt, or sliced banana and low-fat ricotta flavored with honey and ground cinnamon.*

Each serving (2 crepes) provides
427 calories, 17 g protein, 24 g fat (4 g saturated fat), 36 g carbohydrate (8 g sugars), 6 g fiber, 122 mg sodium

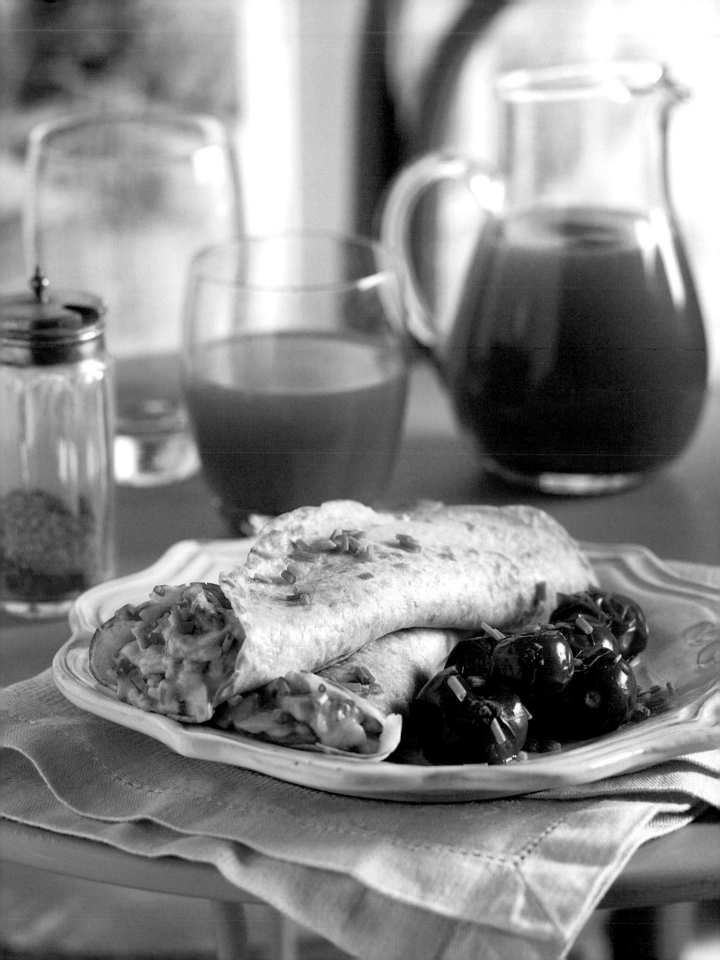

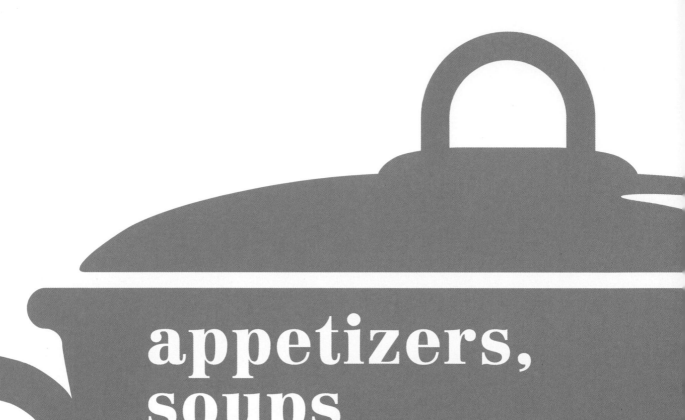

appetizers, soups & sides

chapter 2

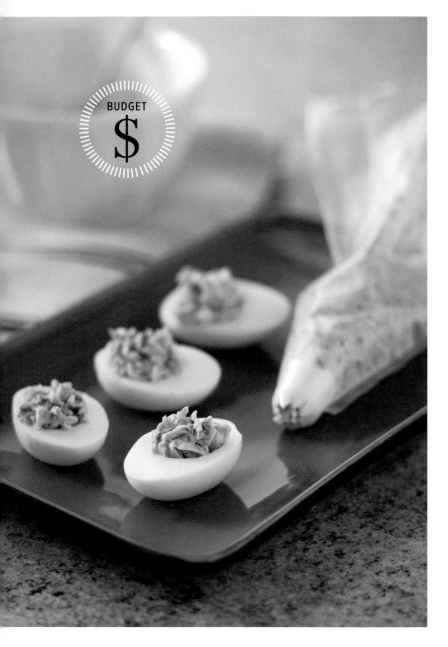

stuffed *eggs*

MAKES 12   PREPARATION 10 MINUTES
COOKING 10 MINUTES

6 hard-boiled eggs
2 tablespoons (30 ml) whole-egg
  mayonnaise
1 teaspoon (5 ml) Dijon mustard
$\frac{1}{4}$ cup (50 g) pimento-stuffed green
  olives, finely chopped
1 small gherkin, finely chopped
1 tablespoon (15 ml) finely chopped
  fresh flat-leaf parsley
freshly ground black pepper

1 Peel each hard-boiled egg and cut
  in half lengthwise. Use a teaspoon
  to carefully remove the egg yolks
  from the whites. Place the yolks in
  a small bowl and mash with a fork.
2 Add the mayonnaise, mustard,
  olives, gherkin and parsley to the
  bowl with the egg yolks and season
  to taste with pepper. Mix to a
  creamy consistency, adding a little
  more mayonnaise if necessary so
  the mixture is moist and light.
3 Pipe or gently spoon the egg yolk
  mixture into each egg-white half,
  mounding it slightly. Refrigerate
  until ready to serve.

Each egg half provides
53 calories, 3 g protein, 4 g fat
(1 g saturated fat), 1 g carbohydrate
(<1 g sugars), <1 g fiber, 149 mg sodium

vegetable *bruschetta*

SERVES 4 PREPARATION 10 MINUTES
COOKING 15 MINUTES

1 red pepper
1 yellow pepper
2 small zucchini
1 bulb fennel
1 red onion
3 tablespoons (45 ml) olive oil
2 cloves garlic
1 small tomato
4 medium slices ciabatta, 1 ounce
  (25 g) each
freshly ground black pepper
12 small fresh basil leaves

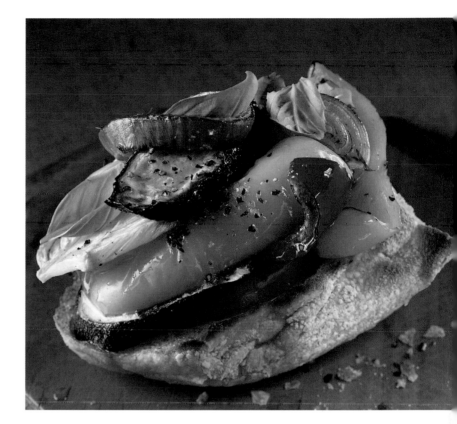

1 Preheat the broiler to high. Cut each pepper lengthwise into eight pieces, and remove the stems and seeds. Trim the zucchini and slice diagonally. Trim the fennel, and cut lengthwise into thin slices. Peel the onion and slice into rings.

2 Arrange the vegetables on a broiler pan in a single layer, positioning the peppers skin sides down. Brush with the oil and broil, on one side only, until lightly browned but still slightly firm. If necessary, cook the vegetables in batches and keep the first batch warm in the oven.

3 Meanwhile, peel and halve the cloves of garlic and halve the tomato. Toast the slices of bread on both sides.

4 Rub the top of each bread slice with the cut garlic and tomato, and pile the grilled vegetables on top. Drizzle the remaining oil over the vegetables and season to taste with pepper. Scatter the basil leaves on top and serve while still warm.

Each serving provides
209 calories, 4 g protein, 15 g fat (2 g saturated fat),
16 g carbohydrate (5 g sugars), 4 g fiber, 139 mg sodium

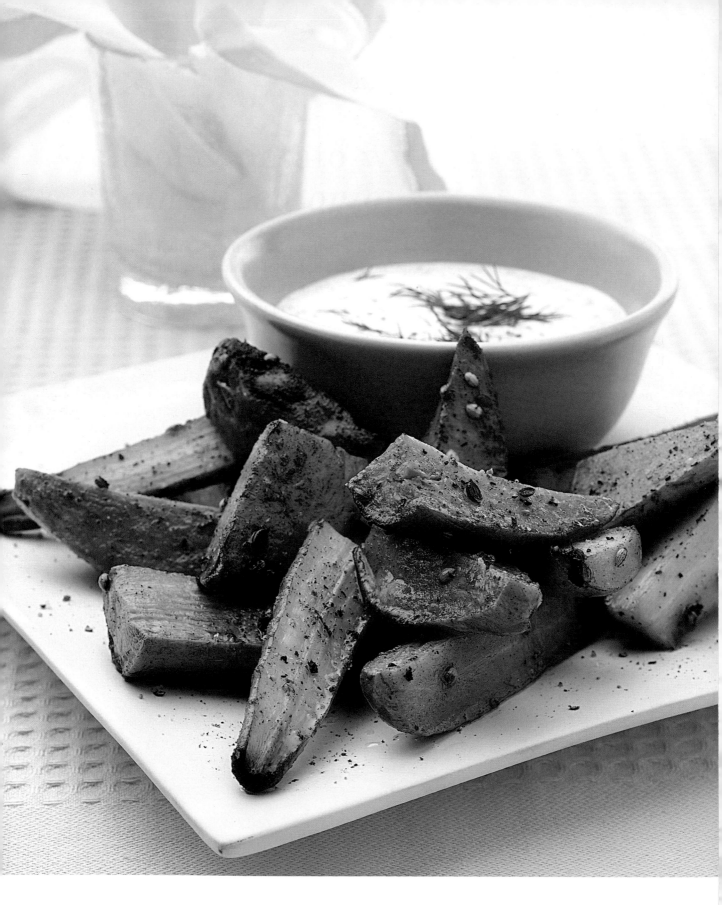

spicy vegetable *wedges*

Here is a lower GI version of potato wedges, made with carrots, parsnips and sweet potatoes. Lightly crushed coriander seeds and a hint of cinnamon accentuate the flavors of the vegetables, which are served with a tangy mustard and yogurt dip.

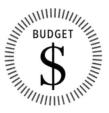
BUDGET
$

SERVES 6   PREPARATION 35 MINUTES   COOKING 40 MINUTES

2 large carrots
2 parsnips
juice of 1 lime
2 tablespoons (30 ml) canola oil
2 tablespoons (30 ml) lightly crushed coriander seeds
$1/2$ teaspoon (2 ml) ground cinnamon
$1/4$ teaspoon (1 ml) freshly ground black pepper
$1^{1/4}$ pounds (600 g) orange sweet potatoes, peeled

Mustard dip
2 teaspoons (10 ml) whole-grain mustard
1 teaspoon (5 ml) superfine sugar
grated zest of 1 lime
1 cup (250 ml) low-fat plain yogurt
3 tablespoons (45 ml) chopped fresh dill, plus extra to garnish

CARROTS, PARSNIPS AND SWEET POTATOES have much less of an effect on blood glucose levels compared to white potatoes, and make an interesting and tasty alternative. To further reduce the GI, use wedges of fresh beets instead of sweet potatoes.

1 Preheat the oven to 425°F (220°C). Cut the carrots and parsnips into wedges. Place them in a saucepan with water to just cover. Bring to a boil, reduce the heat slightly and partially cover the pan. Cook for 2 minutes.
2 Meanwhile, combine the lime juice, oil, coriander, cinnamon and pepper in a roasting pan. Cut the sweet potatoes in half crosswise, then into thick wedges, about the same size as the carrots and parsnips. Add the sweet potatoes to the pan and coat with the spice mixture, and push them to one side of the pan.
3 Drain the carrots and parsnips and add them to the roasting pan. Use a spoon and fork to turn the hot vegetables and coat them with the spice mixture. Place in the oven and roast for 40 minutes, stirring and turning all the vegetables twice, until they are well browned in places and just tender. Remove from the oven and let cool slightly.
4 Meanwhile, to make the mustard dip, combine the mustard, sugar and lime zest in a bowl, and stir in the yogurt and dill. Transfer to a serving bowl, garnish with a little extra dill, and serve with the vegetables.

Each serving provides
171 calories, 5 g protein, 7 g fat (1 g saturated fat),
24 g carbohydrate (11 g sugars), 3 g fiber, 49 mg sodium

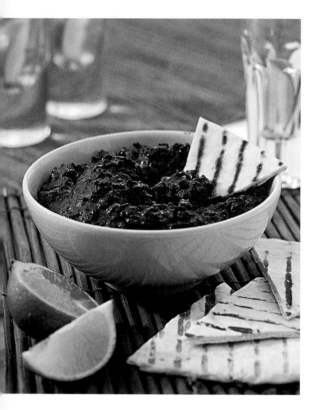

spiced
beet dip

SERVES 4   PREPARATION 15 MINUTES   COOKING 40–60 MINUTES

2 pounds (about 1 kg) beets
1 cup (250 ml) low-fat plain yogurt
2 cloves garlic, crushed
3 tablespoons (45 ml) lemon juice
2 tablespoons (30 ml) extra virgin olive oil
$1/2$ teaspoon (2 ml) ground cumin
$1/2$ teaspoon (2 ml) ground coriander
$1/2$ teaspoon (2 ml) ground cinnamon
$1/2$ teaspoon (2 ml) paprika
freshly ground black pepper

1 Cut off the beet stems about $1/2$ inch (1 cm) from the roots (no closer). Leave the long root at the bottom attached. Scrub the beets very gently but thoroughly, being careful not to break the skin.
2 Cook the beets in a large saucepan of simmering, salted water for 40–60 minutes, or until tender. Drain and allow to cool slightly. When cool enough to handle, rub off the beet skins. It is a good idea to wear rubber gloves when doing this to prevent your hands from becoming stained.
3 Finely chop, grate or process the beets in a food processor, and transfer to a bowl.
4 Add the yogurt to the beets along with the garlic, lemon juice, oil, cumin, coriander, cinnamon and paprika and mix well. Season to taste with pepper. Cover with plastic wrap and refrigerate until required. Serve with warm crusty bread.

Each serving provides
205 calories, 8 g protein, 10 g fat (1 g saturated fat),
22 g carbohydrate (21 g sugars), 7 g fiber, 153 mg sodium

BUDGET
$

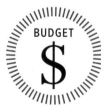

BEETS are very sweet (yet low in calories) and provide significant amounts of vitamin C, folate and potassium. The leafy beet greens are high in calcium and iron.

quinoa with asparagus

SERVES 6   PREPARATION 10 MINUTES
COOKING 15 MINUTES

1 cup (200 g) quinoa, rinsed and
   drained, or brown rice
1 tablespoon (15 ml) olive oil
1 small red onion, thinly sliced
$^{1}/_{2}$ cup (125 ml) homemade or
   low-sodium vegetable
   or chicken stock
$^{3}/_{4}$ pound (400 g) asparagus
   spears, trimmed, cut into
   2 inch (5 cm) pieces
1 cup (150 g) fresh or thawed
   frozen peas
lemon wedges, to serve

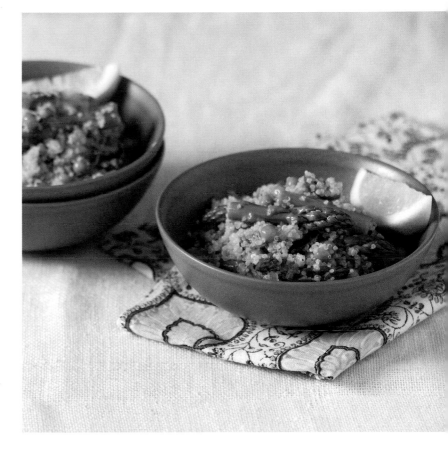

1 Put the quinoa (or brown rice) and
   2 cups (500 ml) water in a small
   saucepan over high heat and bring
   to a boil. Reduce heat to low, cover
   and simmer for 15 minutes, or until
   all the water has been absorbed
   (cook 30 minutes for brown rice).
2 Meanwhile, heat the oil in a large
   nonstick frying pan over medium
   heat. Add the onion and cook for
   about 4 minutes, or until lightly
   browned. Add the stock, asparagus
   and peas and cook for 5 minutes,
   or until just tender.
3 Add the quinoa and stir to mix
   well. Serve immediately with the
   lemon wedges on the side.

Each serving provides
177 calories, 8 g protein, 5 g fat
(3 g saturated fat), 24 g carbohydrate
(2 g sugars), 5 g fiber, 89 mg sodium

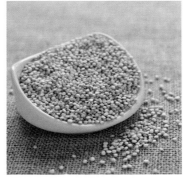

Superfood
   QUINOA contains more
   protein than any other
   grain. Unlike many other
   plant foods, the protein in
   quinoa is complete, in that it
   provides all of the essential
   amino acids, making it the
   perfect grain for vegetarians
   and vegans.

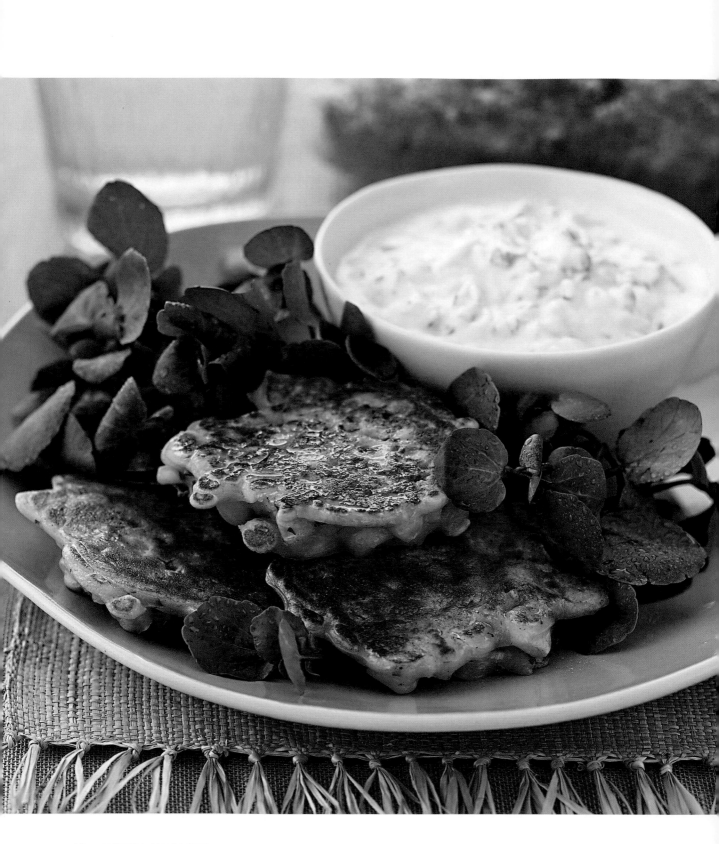

corn *fritters*

These lightly spiced corn fritters served with a minty yogurt sauce make a great summertime starter, or serve them with a salad and whole-grain bread and you've got a great lunch.

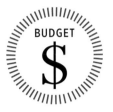

BUDGET
$

SERVES 6 (MAKES 12)   PREPARATION 15 MINUTES   COOKING 15 MINUTES

1 cup (250 ml) low-fat
  Greek-style yogurt
4 scallions, finely chopped
2 tablespoons (30 ml) chopped
  fresh mint
grated zest and juice of 1 lime
3/4 cup (125 g) all-purpose flour
1/2 teaspoon (2 ml) baking powder
1/2 cup (125 ml) low-fat milk
2 eggs, lightly beaten
2 cups (300 g) frozen corn kernels,
  thawed and drained
3 scallions, extra, finely chopped
1 red chile, seeded and
  finely chopped
3 heaping tablespoons (50 ml)
  chopped fresh cilantro leaves
freshly ground black pepper
1 tablespoon (15 ml) canola oil
3 3/4 cups (115 g) watercress, trimmed

1 To make the yogurt sauce, put the yogurt into a serving bowl and stir in the scallions, mint and lime zest (reserve the lime juice for later). Cover and place in the refrigerator to chill while you make the fritters.

2 Sift the flour and baking powder into a mixing bowl. Make a well in the center and add the milk and eggs. Using a wooden spoon, combine the milk and eggs, and gradually draw in the flour from around the edges. Beat with the spoon to make a smooth, thick batter.

3 Add the corn, extra scallions, chile and cilantro to the batter. Season with pepper and stir well.

4 Heat a large heavy-bottom frying pan over medium heat, and brush with a little of the oil. Drop large spoonfuls of the batter onto the pan—make about four fritters at a time—and cook for 2 minutes, or until golden and firm on the underside. Turn the fritters over and cook on the other side for about 2 minutes, or until golden brown.

5 Remove the fritters from the pan and drain on paper towels. Keep warm while cooking the rest of the fritters, adding more oil to the pan as necessary.

6 Arrange the watercress on six plates and sprinkle with the lime juice. Arrange the corn fritters on top and serve hot, with the yogurt sauce on the side.

Each serving (2 fritters) provides
252 calories, 12 g protein, 8 g fat (2 g saturated fat),
33 g carbohydrate (8 g sugars), 4 g fiber, 137 mg sodium

baked tofu squares
with tomato relish

Easy to assemble and a great little snack or starter, this tofu stack will keep the vegetarians happy, too. The relish can be made ahead of time and then heated through just before serving, but the tofu should be cooked close to serving time so it stays crisp.

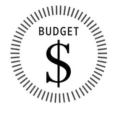

BUDGET

$

SERVES 4   PREPARATION 20 MINUTES   COOKING 25 MINUTES

10 ounces (300 g) firm tofu
2 tablespoons (30 ml)
   all-purpose flour
freshly ground black pepper
1 teaspoon (15 ml) olive oil, for
   brushing

Tomato relish
3 teaspoons (15 ml) olive oil
1 small onion, finely chopped
1 teaspoon (5 ml) ground coriander
1/2 teaspoon (2 ml) ground cumin
1/2 teaspoon (2 ml) mild paprika
1 1/3 cups (350 g) ripe tomatoes,
   finely chopped
2 teaspoons (10 ml) balsamic
   vinegar
1/4 cup (15 g) chopped fresh cilantro
   leaves and stems

1 Preheat the oven to 425°F (220°C). Line a baking pan with parchment paper. Drain the tofu on a few layers of folded paper towel and leave for about 5 minutes to remove the surface moisture.

2 Meanwhile, make the tomato relish. Heat the oil in a saucepan over medium heat, add the onion and cook, stirring, for 4 minutes, or until soft. Add the ground coriander, cumin and paprika and cook, stirring, for 30 seconds. Add the tomatoes and any tomato juices, along with the vinegar. Bring to a simmer, and cook, uncovered, stirring frequently, for 20 minutes, or until thick. Stir in the chopped cilantro. Remove the pan from the heat and cover to keep warm.

3 Meanwhile, cut the tofu into 1/2 inch (1 cm) slices, and halve each slice crosswise. Combine the flour and pepper on a plate. Toss the tofu pieces in the flour mixture to coat lightly. Place them on the baking pan and brush with oil. Bake for 25 minutes, or until pale golden on the edges.

4 Stack three pieces of warm tofu on top of each other, and top with a spoonful of tomato relish. If you like, use toothpicks to secure the tofu stacks.

Each serving provides
164 calories, 11 g protein, 10 g fat (1 g saturated fat),
8 g carbohydrate (3 g sugars), 3 g fiber, 16 mg sodium

THIS SNACK OF TOFU, topped with a richly spiced tomato relish, combines the benefits of soy protein with the cancer-protecting properties of cooked tomato and the strong antioxidant substances in cumin, cilantro and paprika.

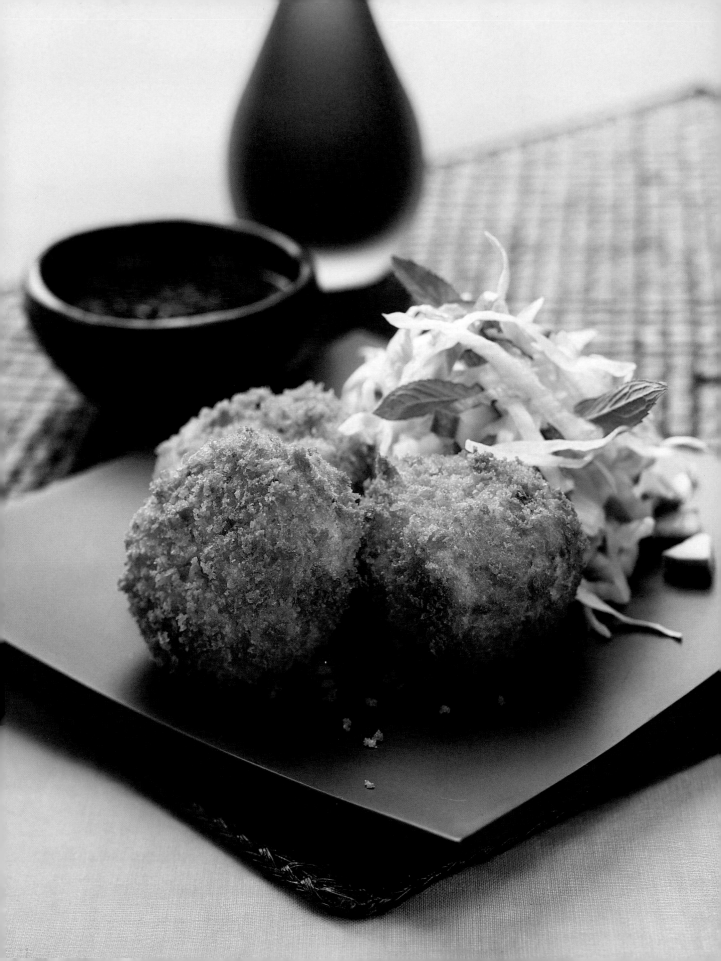

thai *fish cakes*

These delicious fish cakes, made with fresh fish and potatoes, are flavored with lemongrass and cilantro, and spiced with Thai red curry paste. Served with a lettuce, cucumber and mint salad, they make a tempting starter.

SERVES 12 (MAKES 24)   PREPARATION 20 MINUTES, PLUS 1 HOUR CHILLING   COOKING 35 MINUTES

$2/3$ pound (350 g) russet potatoes, peeled and chopped

$2/3$ pound (350 g) firm white fish fillets

juice of 1 lime

2 teaspoons (10 ml) Thai red curry paste

1 thin lemongrass stem, white only, thinly sliced, lightly crushed

3 scallions, thinly sliced

3 cloves garlic, chopped

$1/4$ cup (15 g) chopped fresh cilantro leaves

1 teaspoon (5 ml) finely chopped fresh ginger

pinch of salt

$1/3$ cup (50 g) all-purpose flour

2 eggs, lightly beaten

$1 1/4$ cups (100 g) fresh breadcrumbs

2 tablespoons (30 ml) extra virgin olive oil

Salad

1 butter lettuce, finely shredded

$1/2$ cucumber, diced

$3/4$ cup (15 g) fresh mint leaves

Each serving (2 fish cakes) provides
142 calories, 10 g protein, 5 g fat
(1 g saturated fat), 14 g carbohydrate
(1 g sugars), 2 g fiber, 153 mg sodium

1 Put the potatoes in a saucepan and add enough boiling water to cover by 2 inches (5 cm). Bring to a boil, reduce heat and cook for 15–20 minutes, or until tender. Drain into a large bowl and mash.

2 While the potatoes are cooking, put the fish in a shallow pan with enough cold water to cover and add half of the lime juice. Bring to a boil, reduce the heat to low and simmer for 1 minute. Remove from the heat, cover the pan and let the fish cool in the liquid for about 4 minutes. Drain the fish and flake the flesh with a fork, discarding the skin and any bones.

3 Add the fish to the potatoes in the bowl and combine well with a fork, adding the curry paste, lemongrass, scallions, garlic, cilantro, ginger and the remaining lime juice. Season with the salt.

4 Put the flour on a plate. Pour the eggs into a shallow bowl. Sprinkle the breadcrumbs on another plate. Take about 1 tablespoon (15 ml) of the fish mixture and shape it into a small fish cake. Roll the cake in flour, shaking off the excess, then dip into the egg and, finally, coat with crumbs, turning and pressing on the crumbs to coat all sides evenly. Shape and coat the remaining fish cakes in the same way, making 24 in total. Cover and refrigerate for 1 hour.

5 Heat half of the oil in a large nonstick frying pan over medium heat. Add half of the fish cakes and cook for about 3 minutes on each side, or until lightly golden and crisp. Remove and keep warm while you cook the rest of the fish cakes, using the remaining oil.

6 Meanwhile, to make the salad, combine the lettuce, cucumber and mint in a bowl. Arrange the fish cakes on individual plates with the salad and serve.

citrus-marinated *scallops*

This quick-and-easy dish is a good source of omega-3s, as well as antioxidants, thanks to the citrus and herbs. The scallops are best pan-fried over a fairly high heat, as this gives them a golden crust and seals in their juices.

SERVES 4   PREPARATION 15 MINUTES   COOKING 5 MINUTES

1 lime
1 small lemon
2 small oranges
2 tablespoons (30 ml) extra virgin
   olive oil
12 large fresh scallops, without roe
1 cup (30 g) fresh cilantro leaves
1 cup (30 g) watercress sprigs,
   trimmed
freshly ground black pepper

1 Finely grate the zest of the lime, lemon and 1 orange. Put the citrus zest and 1 tablespoon (15 ml) of the oil in a bowl and combine. Add the scallops and gently stir to coat well with the marinade.
2 Discard the white pith from the lemon and both oranges, and carefully cut out the segments with a sharp knife. Slice each lemon segment into two or three pieces. Leave the orange segments whole. Put the lemon and orange segments in a serving bowl, and add the cilantro leaves and watercress sprigs.
3 Juice the lime and pour into a small bowl. Add the remaining oil and a little pepper and whisk together. Set the dressing aside.
4 Heat a large nonstick frying pan over medium–high heat. Add the scallops and cook for 1–2 minutes on each side. Remove the scallops from the heat and gently toss with the lemon and orange segments, cilantro and watercress. Pour the dressing over all and toss gently to combine. Serve immediately.

Each serving provides
132 calories, 6 g protein, 10 g fat (1 g saturated fat),
6 g carbohydrate (5 g sugars), 2 g fiber, 73 mg sodium

Frozen scallops can be used for this recipe. Thaw overnight in the refrigerator, pat dry with paper towels and marinate as in step 1.

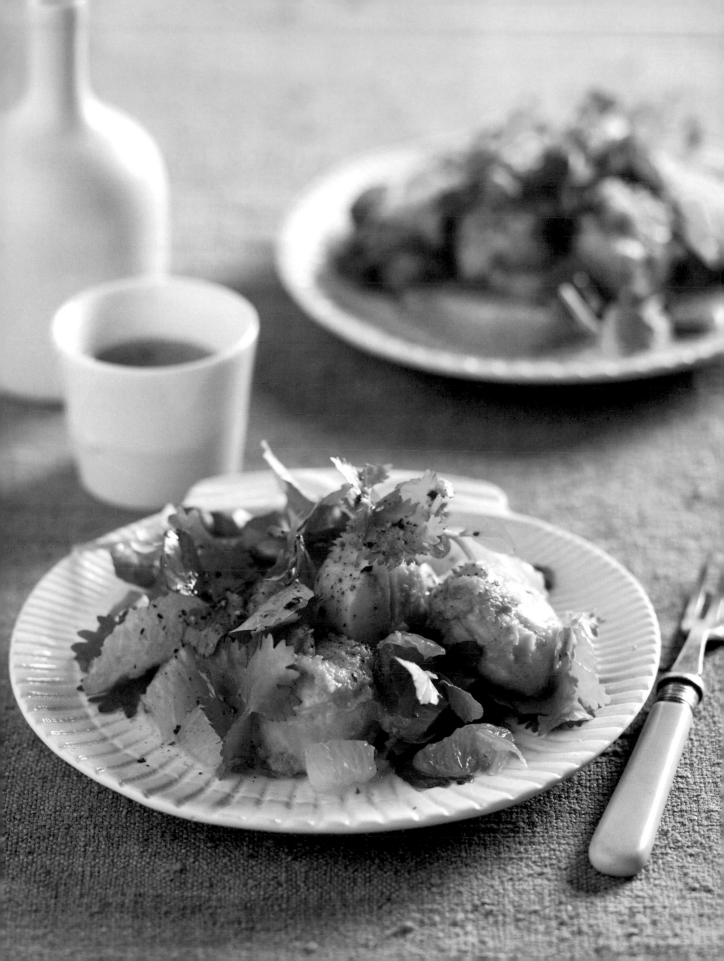

fresh fruit *soup*

Not only is this refreshing soup perfect on a sweltering summer day, it could also give you a vitamin boost in winter. Made with a variety of vitamin-packed raw fruits and vegetables, it has a low GI and is an easy way to load up on protective nutrients.

SERVES 4   PREPARATION 30 MINUTES, PLUS 1 HOUR CHILLING   COOKING NONE

1 cup (250 ml) unsweetened
   pineapple juice
2 cups (500 ml) unsweetened
   orange juice
$^1/_2$ cucumber, diced
$^1/_4$ red onion, finely chopped
1 small red pepper, seeded
   and chopped
$^1/_2$ red chile, seeded and chopped
juice of 1 lime
$^1/_2$ teaspoon (2 ml) superfine sugar
1 large mango
10 white grapes
1 firm pear
2 passion fruit
1 tablespoon (15 ml) chopped
   fresh mint
2 tablespoons (30 ml) chopped
   fresh cilantro leaves
sprigs of fresh mint, to garnish

1 Combine the pineapple juice, orange juice and 1 cup (250 ml) water in a large bowl. Add the cucumber, onion, pepper, chile, lime juice and sugar and stir well. Cover and place in the refrigerator to chill for 1 hour, to allow the flavors to develop.

2 Cut and dice the mango flesh and add to the soup. Halve the grapes and core and dice the pear, then add to the soup. Cut the passion fruit in half, scoop out the flesh with a teaspoon and stir into the soup. Add the chopped mint and cilantro.

3 Ladle the soup into bowls and garnish with mint sprigs. Serve at once.

ANOTHER IDEA

+ *Purée the soup (without the passion fruit pulp) in a blender or food processor to make a vitamin-packed refreshing drink any time of year.*

Each serving provides
148 calories, 3 g protein, 1 g fat (0 g saturated fat),
33 g carbohydrate (30 g sugars), 5 g fiber, 20 mg sodium

HEALTHY EATING Nutritionists recommend a daily quota of seven or more servings of fruits and vegetables for optimum health and well-being. This soup is a great way to help you meet this target.

STUDIES into the incidence of bowel cancer within different population groups suggest that people who eat more fruits and vegetables are less likely to get this disease.

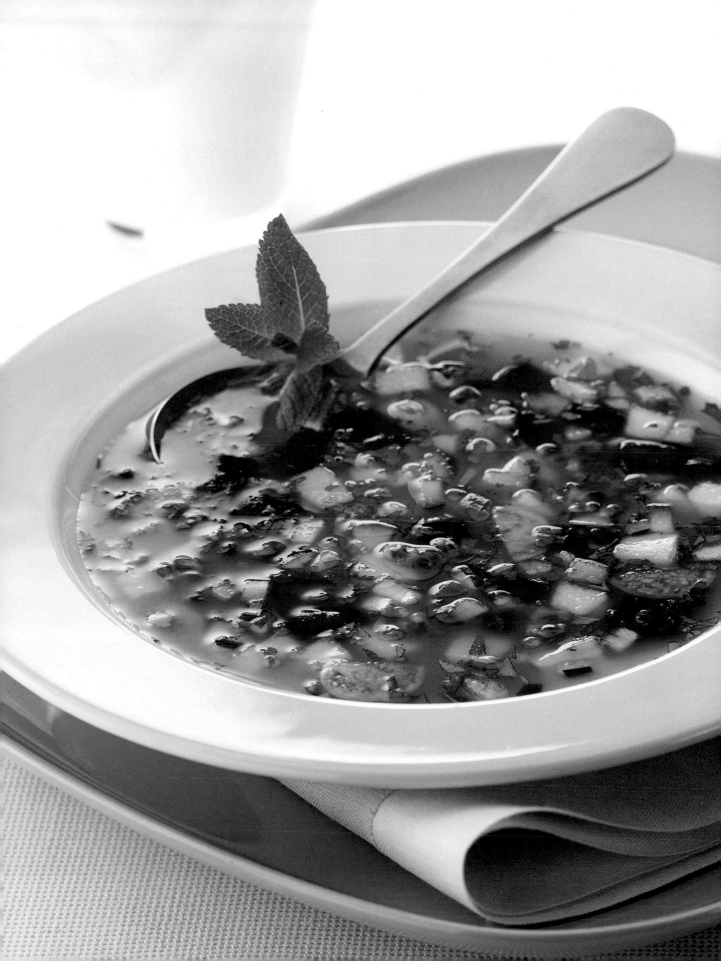

beet & *cranberry borscht*

Cranberry juice brings sweetness and fruity goodness to red cabbage and purple beets in a soup that is full of vitamins and antioxidants. For a main meal, serve with whole-grain bread.

SERVES 6   PREPARATION 10 MINUTES   COOKING 15 MINUTES

1 tablespoon (15 ml) olive oil
1 onion, chopped
2 celery stalks, chopped
2 cloves garlic, crushed
$1/2$ teaspoon (2 ml) ground mace
   or nutmeg
$1/2$ teaspoon (2 ml) ground allspice
$1^1/4$ cups (300 g) red cabbage, finely
   shredded
$2/3$ cup (150 ml) chicken stock, hot
$2^1/2$ cups (600 ml) cranberry
   juice drink
$1^3/4$ cups (450 g) cooked beets, diced
2 teaspoons (10 ml) red wine
   vinegar or cider vinegar
2 tablespoons (30 ml) lemon juice
freshly ground black pepper
4 tablespoons (60 ml) low-fat
   plain yogurt
3 tablespoons (45 ml) snipped chives

1 Heat the oil in a large saucepan over high heat, add the onion, celery, garlic, mace and allspice and stir to combine. Reduce the heat to medium, then cover the pan and cook for 4 minutes, or until the vegetables begin to soften.

2 Add the cabbage to the pan and cook, stirring, for 1 minute. Add the hot stock, $1^3/4$ cups (450 ml) water and the cranberry juice drink. Stir in the beets and bring to a boil. Reduce the heat to low, cover and cook at a slow simmer for 10 minutes.

3 Stir in the vinegar and lemon juice and season to taste with pepper. Ladle the soup into four bowls, then top each serving with 1 tablespoon (15 ml) yogurt and sprinkle with chives.

Each serving provides
141 calories, 4 g protein, 4 g fat (<1 g saturated fat), 23 g carbohydrate (22 g sugars), 5 g fiber, 148 mg sodium

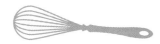

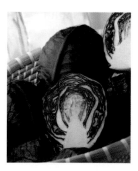

Superfood
RED CABBAGE belongs to the brassica family, with broccoli and watercress. It is bursting with antioxidant nutrients, and provides vitamin C and B vitamins, such as folate. Evidence links brassicas with a reduced risk for cancer of the digestive tract.

Cut the cabbage into short fine shreds by slicing it into slim wedges and then finely slicing the wedges—the cabbage should then fall apart.

Vacuum-packed cooked beets are a brilliant pantry ingredient with a long shelf life. For this recipe, make sure it is not the kind preserved with vinegar. Otherwise, boil or bake unpeeled beets until tender, rub off the skins, and use as directed above.

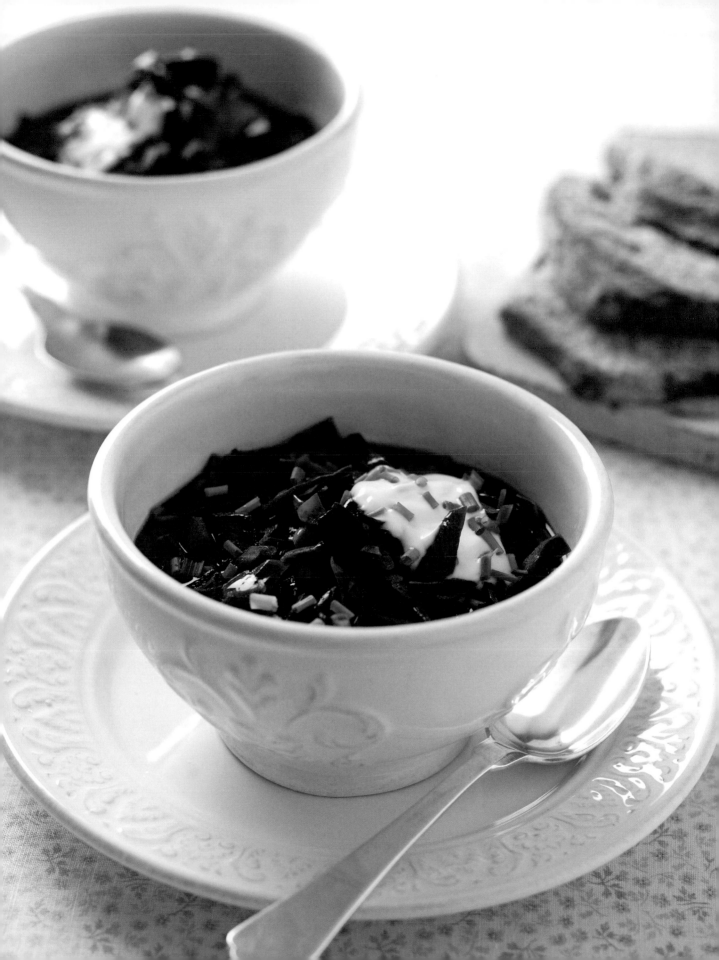

oven-baked potato wedges

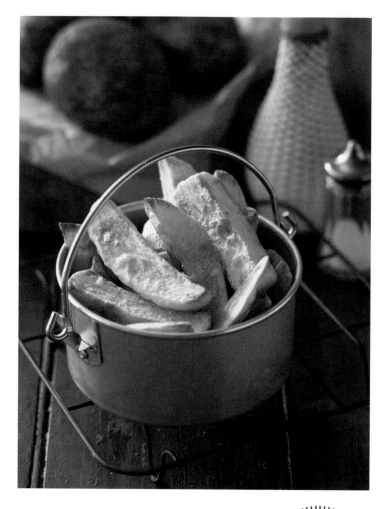

SERVES 4   PREPARATION 10 MINUTES
COOKING 40 MINUTES

1 tablespoon (15 ml) olive oil
3 large roasting potatoes, such as
   russet or Yukon gold, about
   1^1/$_2$ pounds (750 g)
pinch of salt

1 Preheat the oven to 400F (200°C).
   Lightly grease a baking tray
   with 1 teaspoon (5 ml) of the oil.
2 Wash and peel the potatoes, then
   cut into wedges about ^{3}/$_4$ inch
   (1.5 cm) thick. Place the wedges in
   a clean dish towel and pat dry.
3 Spread the wedges on the baking
   tray, drizzle with the remaining
   oil and toss to coat. Bake for
   40 minutes, or until golden brown,
   turning occasionally. Season with
   salt and serve hot.

ANOTHER IDEA

+ *Russet potatoes make great potato
   wedges. Don't bother peeling them,
   just cut them lengthwise into thick
   wedges and toss in olive oil. Bake for
   40 minutes, or until golden brown.*

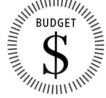

BUDGET
$

Each serving provides
163 calories, 5 g protein, 5 g fat
(1 g saturated fat), 25 g carbohydrate
(1 g sugars), 3 g fiber, 78 mg sodium

potato *latkes*

SERVES 6 (MAKES 12)   PREPARATION
20 MINUTES   COOKING 20 MINUTES

2 pounds (1 kg) potatoes, such as
   russet, peeled
1 small onion, finely chopped
2 eggs, lightly beaten
1/3 cup (50 g) all-purpose flour
1 teaspoon (5 ml) baking powder
1 tablespoon (15 ml) vegetable oil,
   for pan-frying

1 Grate the potatoes into a bowl, and
   combine with the onion. Take a handful
   of the mixture and squeeze over a bowl
   to remove as much liquid as possible.
   Place the mixture into a clean bowl.
2 Add the eggs, and sift in the flour and
   baking powder. Combine well.
3 Heat about 1/4 inch (0.5 cm) of oil in a
   large heavy-bottom frying pan over
   medium heat. Drop 1/3 cups (75 ml) of
   the mixture into the pan, and flatten to
   3 inches (8 cm). You should be able to
   cook three or four at a time, but don't
   crowd the pan. Cook for 3 minutes on
   each side, or until brown and crisp.
4 Drain on paper towels and keep warm
   while you cook the remaining latkes.
   Serve hot.

ANOTHER IDEA

+ *You could make smaller latkes and
   top them with a little smoked salmon
   and a small spoonful of sour cream.*

Each serving provides
190 calories, 7 g protein, 5 g fat
(1 g saturated fat), 28 g carbohydrate
(1 g sugars), 3 g fiber, 67 mg sodium

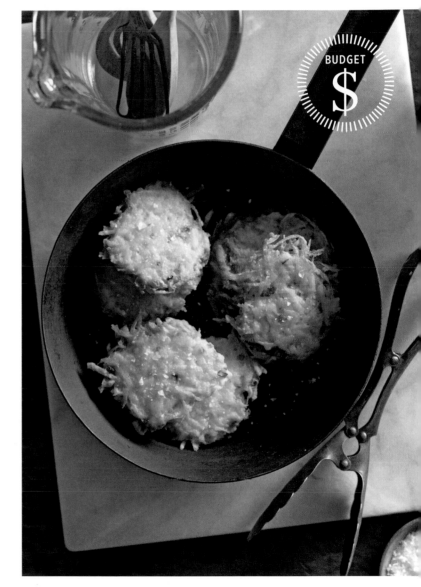

BUDGET
$

butternut squash with *peppers & almonds*

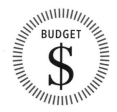

BUDGET
$

This sunny medley of vitamin-rich butternut squash and yellow peppers is tossed in a nut-and-honey glaze. It's ideal as a side dish or serve it as a vegetarian main course with whole-grain bread.

SERVES 4   PREPARATION 10 MINUTES   COOKING 20 MINUTES

1¼ pounds (600 g) butternut squash
3 teaspoons (15 ml) olive oil
2 cloves garlic, thinly sliced
8 sprigs fresh thyme
2 yellow peppers
¼ cup (50 g) whole almonds
1 tablespoon (15 ml) honey
finely grated zest and juice
    of 1 lemon

1 Preheat the oven to 400°F (200°C). Peel the squash and scoop out the seeds. Cut the squash into 12 slices, each about ½ inch (1 cm) thick. Transfer the slices to a shallow roasting pan. Drizzle the squash with 2 teaspoons (10 ml) of the oil and add the garlic and thyme. Roast for 20 minutes, or until softened and beginning to brown.

2 Meanwhile, slice the peppers into ½ inch (1 cm) strips. When the squash has just 5 minutes of cooking time left, heat the remaining 1 teaspoon (5 ml) oil in a frying pan over medium–high heat. Add the pepper strips and fry for 5 minutes, stirring frequently, until they are tender and beginning to brown. Transfer the peppers and squash to a warmed serving dish.

3 Add the almonds, honey, lemon zest and lemon juice to the frying pan. Stir-fry over high heat for a few seconds until the mixture is bubbling and the lemon juice and honey have thickened to form a glaze. Spoon the honey glaze over the vegetables and serve.

Each serving provides
193 calories, 4 g protein, 10 g fat (1 g saturated fat),
23 g carbohydrate (11 g sugars), 4 g fiber, 7 mg sodium

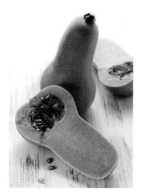

Superfood
    BUTTERNUT SQUASH is an excellent source of both soluble and insoluble fiber, and a low-GI food. The nutrient-packed orange flesh is bursting with antioxidants alpha- and beta-carotene, as well as vitamins C and E.

Butternut squash will continue to soften after it has been removed from the oven. To test for doneness, carefully prick with a fork—it should be tender but firm.

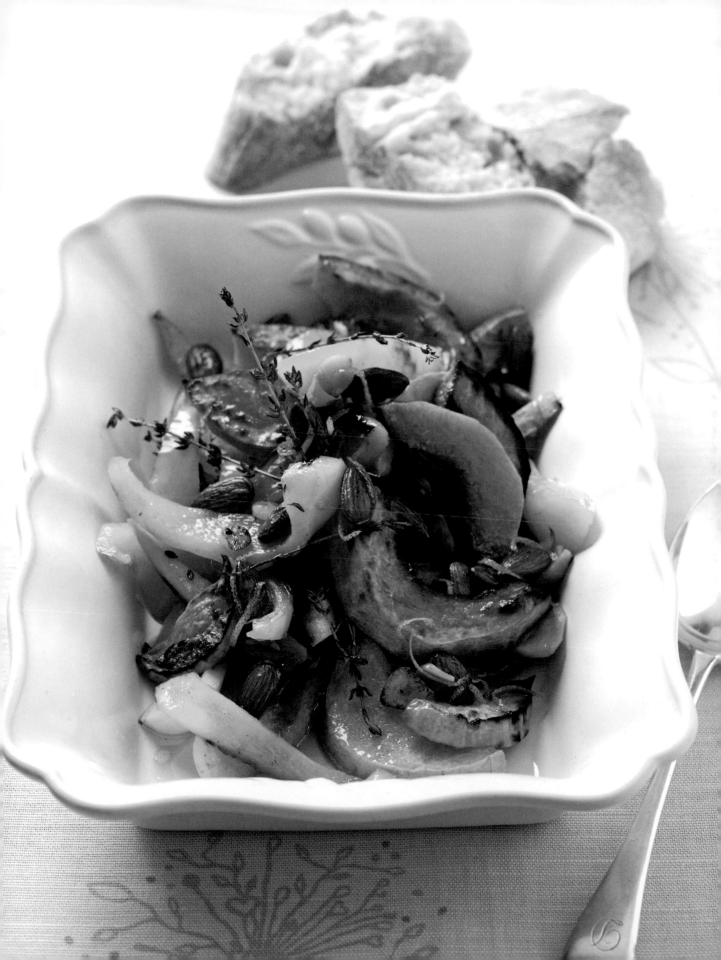

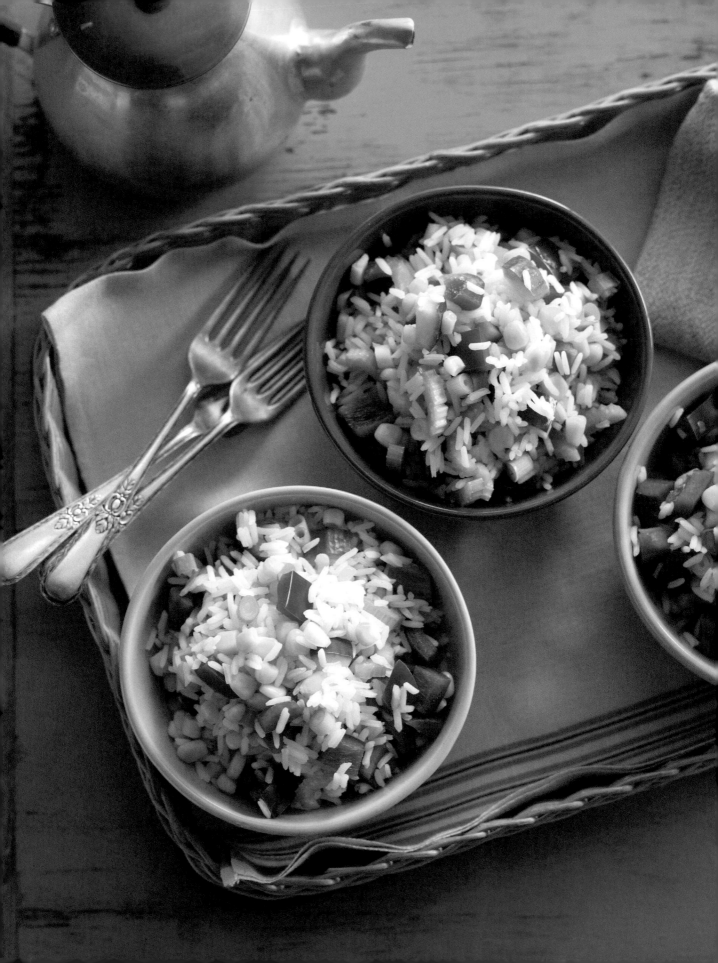

rice *salad*

Rice salads are easy to prepare, especially if you have some cooked rice left over from the night before. Just about any vegetable will work well, so don't feel bound by what's listed here. Rice salad is the perfect partner for grilled or barbecued chicken or fish.

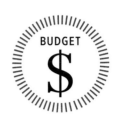

BUDGET
$

SERVES 8   PREPARATION 15 MINUTES   COOKING 10 MINUTES

1 cup (250 g) long-grain
   white rice
1¼ cups (300 g) canned
   corn kernels, drained
4 scallions, sliced
1 small red pepper, seeded
   and diced
1 small cucumber, diced
2 celery stalks, sliced
3 tablespoons (45 ml) lemon juice
2 tablespoons (30 ml) olive oil

1 Cook the rice in a large saucepan of boiling water for 10 minutes, or until just tender. Drain well. Let cool, turning the rice over occasionally with a large metal spoon to release the heat.

2 Once the rice has cooled to room temperature, fold in all the vegetables. Whisk together the lemon juice and oil, pour over the rice and fold in to combine. Serve immediately at room temperature, or cover and refrigerate until ready to serve.

ANOTHER IDEA
+ *Add some cubed pineapple, quartered cherry tomatoes or a handful of roasted chopped cashews to the rice.*

Each serving provides
160 calories, 3 g protein, 5 g fat (1 g saturated fat), 26 g carbohydrate (2 g sugars), 2 g fiber, 78 mg sodium

Rice left unrefrigerated can pose a food poisoning risk. If not using it immediately, keep the rice covered in the refrigerator. Take the rice out 20 minutes before serving to take off the chill.

ratatouille

Traditionally, the vegetables for a ratatouille are cooked separately and the dish is assembled at the end. This method is quicker but the results are just as tasty.

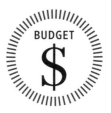

BUDGET $

SERVES 6   PREPARATION 20 MINUTES   COOKING 35 MINUTES

2 tablespoons (30 ml) olive oil
1 onion, chopped
2 cloves garlic, crushed
1 red pepper, seeded and cut
   into 1 inch (2.5 cm) pieces
2 zucchini, cut in half lengthwise,
   and into 1 inch (2.5 cm) slices
1 eggplant, cut into 1 inch
   (2.5 cm) cubes
5 ripe tomatoes, cored and chopped
2 tablespoons (30 ml) shredded fresh
   basil, plus extra leaves to garnish
freshly ground black pepper

1 Heat the oil in a large heavy-bottom saucepan over medium heat. Add the onion and sauté for 7 minutes, or until soft and golden, then add the garlic and cook for another 1 minute.

2 Add the pepper and cook for 2 minutes, stirring occasionally, add the zucchini and eggplant and stir until well combined.

3 Stir in the tomatoes and bring to a boil. Reduce the heat to low and partially cover. Simmer, stirring occasionally, for 20 minutes, or until the vegetables are tender. Stir in the basil and season to taste with pepper. Serve hot or warm, with extra basil leaves scattered on each serving.

ANOTHER IDEA
+ *To make a vegetarian main meal, add a drained and rinsed 14^1/$_2$ ounce (400 gram) can of chickpeas at the end of cooking and heat through. Serve with crusty bread.*

Each serving provides
94 calories, 3 g protein, 7 g fat (1 g saturated fat),
6 g carbohydrate (5 g sugars), 4 g fiber, 13 mg sodium

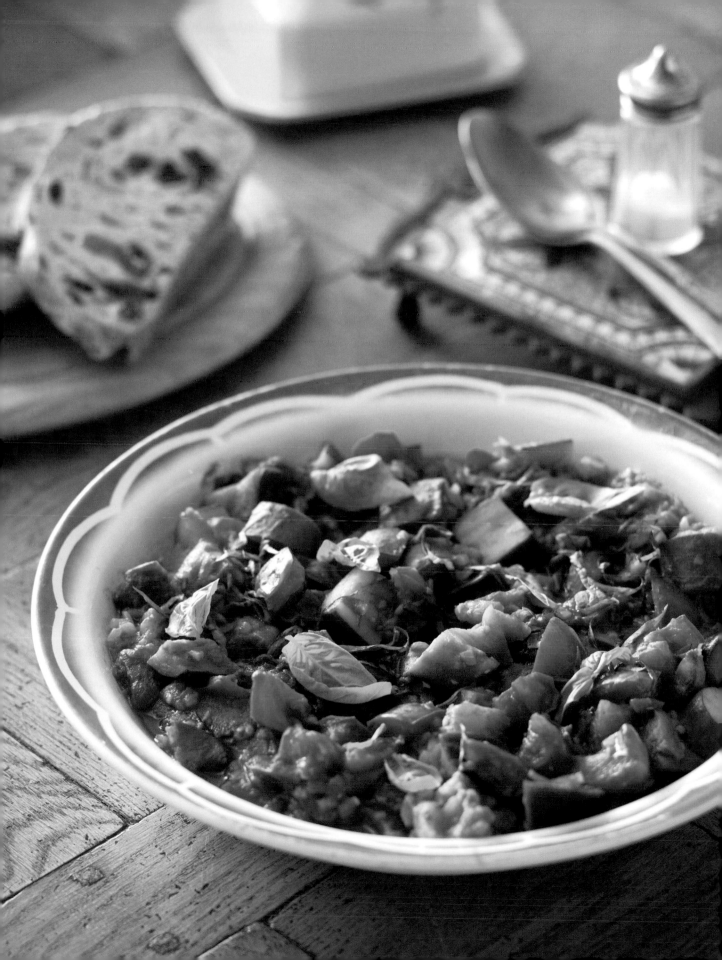

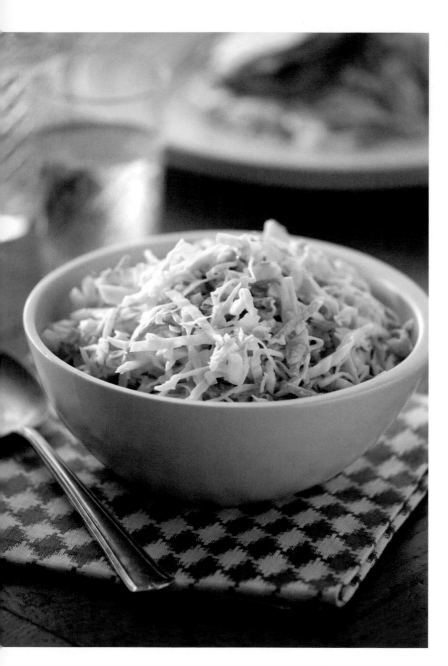

coleslaw

SERVES 8   PREPARATION 15 MINUTES
COOKING NONE

$1/4$ small head of green cabbage
1 large carrot, coarsely grated
1 small red onion, finely chopped
$1/4$ cup (60 ml) good-quality
   mayonnaise, such as
   whole-egg mayonnaise
2 tablespoons (30 ml) lemon juice

1 Discard any damaged outer leaves
from the cabbage. Using a large
sharp knife, shred the cabbage as
finely as possible, discarding any
thick ribs. Place in a large bowl
and toss with the carrot and onion.
2 Combine the mayonnaise and
lemon juice. Add to the vegetables
and toss to combine. Serve
immediately, or cover and
refrigerate until needed.

OTHER IDEAS
+ *Replace the lemon juice with
white wine vinegar if you don't
have a lemon.*
+ *Replace green cabbage with red
cabbage or a combination of red and
green, and use 4 thinly sliced
scallions instead of the red onion.*
+ *For extra kick, add 2 teaspoons
(10 ml) whole-grain or Dijon mustard
to the dressing.*

Each serving provides
62 calories, 1 g protein, 6 g fat
(1 g saturated fat), 1 g carbohydrate
(1 g sugars), 1 g fiber, 10 mg sodium

glazed *carrots*

SERVES 6   PREPARATION 10 MINUTES
COOKING 10 MINUTES

3 carrots
1 tablespoon (20 ml) butter
1 tablespoon (15 ml) honey

1 Peel the carrots and cut into
$1/4$-inch (0.5-cm) slices on a slight
diagonal. Cook in a saucepan of
boiling water over medium heat for
5 minutes, or until just tender.
Drain off the water; return the pan
and carrots to the stovetop.

2 Add the butter and honey to the
pan. Cook over low heat, stirring
and tossing, for about 2 minutes,
or until the carrots are well glazed,
and serve.

ANOTHER IDEA

+ *For a special occasion, use a bunch of*
whole baby carrots instead. Trim the
tops, leaving about $3/4$ inch (1.5 cm) of
green stalk, then peel and cook as
directed. Add a little chopped fresh
parsley or a pinch of ground cumin to
the honey glaze, if desired.

Each serving provides
46 calories, <1 g protein, 3 g fat
(2 g saturated fat), 6 g carbohydrate
(5 g sugars), 1 g fiber, 37 mg sodium

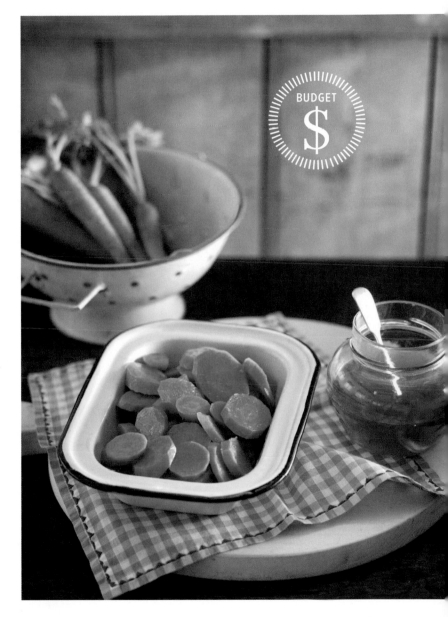

BUDGET
$

vegetarian, salads & pasta

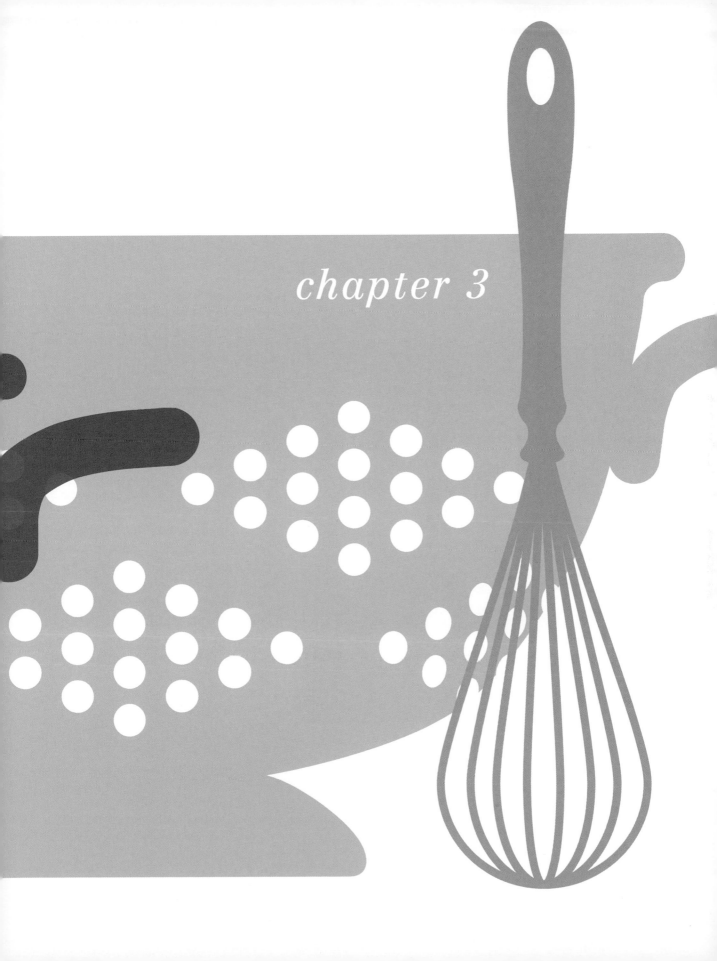

chapter 3

fresh rice paper rolls

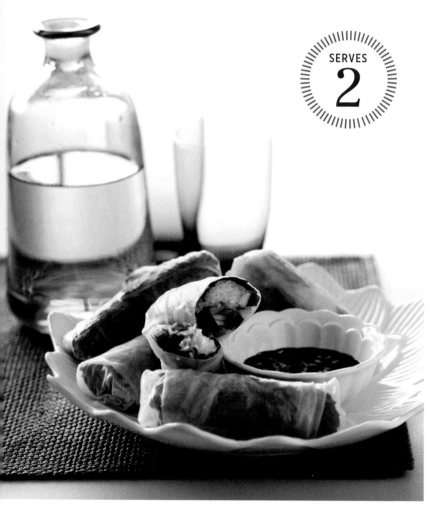

SERVES 2

SERVES 2 (MAKES 6)
PREPARATION 15 MINUTES   COOKING NONE

$\frac{1}{4}$ cup (50 g) rice vermicelli noodles
1 red pepper
1 carrot
1 cucumber, seeds removed
10 snow peas
2 scallions
6 round rice paper wrappers
6 fresh mint or basil leaves
6 cilantro leaves

Dipping sauce
1 tablespoon (15 ml) hoisin sauce
2 teaspoons (10 ml) low-sodium
  soy sauce
drop of sesame oil
1 teaspoon (5 ml) crushed nuts

1 Put the noodles in a heatproof bowl.
  Cover with boiling water and soak
  for 6–8 minutes, or until softened.
  Drain, then cut into shorter lengths.
2 Meanwhile, slice the vegetables into
  long, thin strips. To make the dipping
  sauce, combine the ingredients in a
  small bowl.
3 Working with one sheet at a time,
  place a rice paper wrapper in a bowl
  of warm water for about 30 seconds,
  or until softened. Place on a clean
  board and pat dry with a paper towel.
4 Arrange some of the noodles,
  vegetables and herbs in the center of
  the rice paper wrapper. Fold one side
  of the wrapper over to partially cover
  the filling, fold in the two sides, then
  continue rolling to form a cigar
  shape, enclosing the filling. Repeat
  with the remaining wrappers and
  filling ingredients. Serve with the
  dipping sauce.

Each serving (3 rolls) provides
283 calories, 6 g protein, 3 g fat
(<1 g saturated fat), 58 g carbohydrate
(11 g sugars), 5 g fiber, 452 mg sodium

bulgur & shrimp salad

SERVES 4   PREPARATION 15 MINUTES
COOKING 15 MINUTES

1^1/$_2$ cups (265 g) bulgur
1 small red onion, very thinly sliced
1 carrot, coarsely grated
1 tomato, diced
6 baby corn, sliced into rounds
^{1}/$_2$ cucumber, diced
^{1}/$_2$ pound (250 g) peeled cooked shrimp

Lime and chile dressing
^{1}/$_3$ cup (75 ml) extra virgin olive oil
2 tablespoons (30 ml) lime juice
1 clove garlic, crushed
^{1}/$_4$ teaspoon (1 ml) dried red chile flakes
pinch of salt
freshly ground black pepper

1 Put the bulgur in a saucepan and cover
  with 2^1/$_2$ cups (625 ml) water. Bring to a
  boil, and simmer for 10 minutes, or until
  the bulgur is tender and all the water
  is absorbed. Put the bulgur on a plate,
  spread it out and allow to cool slightly.
2 Combine the onion, carrot, tomato, corn,
  cucumber and shrimp in a large salad
  bowl. Add the bulgur and mix together.
3 To make the dressing, put all the
  ingredients in a small bowl and stir
  well to combine. Before serving, add the
  dressing to the salad, tossing to coat all
  the ingredients evenly.

Each serving provides
447 calories, 19 g protein, 20 g fat
(3 g saturated fat), 44 g carbohydrate
(3 g sugars), 10 g fiber, 383 mg sodium

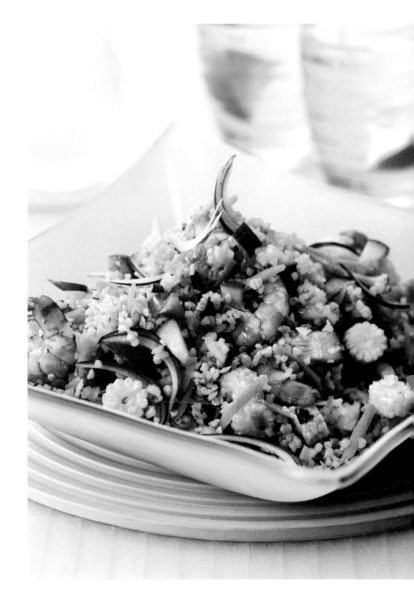

BULGUR is a low-GI carbohydrate and a good source
of dietary fiber and B vitamins It contains all the
nutritious outer layers of the grain except the bran itself.

USING THE RAW VEGETABLES in this salad
not only adds texture and color but also vitamins,
particularly those with antioxidant properties.

SHRIMP, like all shellfish, contain iodine, which is
needed for the production of thyroid hormones
and the normal functioning of the thyroid gland.

bulgur & fish salad
with lemon dressing

This is a variation on the classic and much-loved Middle Eastern tabbouleh. Fresh cilantro, mint and parsley are a trifecta of antioxidant rich, vitamin-packed herbs, and the addition of fish takes this from a side dish to a healthy, protein-powered main course.

SERVES 4   PREPARATION 15 MINUTES, PLUS 45 MINUTES SOAKING AND 1–2 HOURS CHILLING   COOKING 10 MINUTES

1 cup (175 g) bulgur
²/₃ pound (300 g) boneless, skinless firm white fish fillets
1 small lemon, thinly sliced
2 sprigs parsley
5 black peppercorns
1 cucumber, seeds removed, diced
4 scallions, thinly sliced
1 cup (250 g) cherry tomatoes, halved
2 tablespoons (30 ml) chopped fresh cilantro leaves
2 tablespoons (30 ml) chopped fresh mint, plus mint sprigs, to garnish
2 tablespoons (30 ml) chopped fresh parsley

Lemon dressing
2 tablespoons (30 ml) olive oil
2 tablespoons (30 ml) red wine vinegar
2 tablespoons (30 ml) lemon juice
1 tablespoon (15 ml) finely grated lemon zest
1 teaspoon (5 ml) Dijon mustard
1 clove garlic, crushed
pinch of salt
freshly ground black pepper, to taste

1 Put the bulgur in a heatproof bowl and cover with 2 cups (500 ml) boiling water. Set aside for 45 minutes, or until the grains are tender and the water has been absorbed.

2 Meanwhile, place the fish fillets in a large saucepan, add the lemon slices, parsley sprigs and peppercorns, and add enough cold water to cover. Bring to a boil, reduce the heat and simmer, covered, for 5 minutes, or until the fish is opaque and flakes easily. Remove the fish from the liquid and set aside to cool. Use a fork to separate the fish into large flakes.

3 Place the bulgur in a serving bowl and add the cucumber, scallions, tomatoes and chopped herbs. Gently mix in the fish, taking care not to break it up.

4 To make the lemon dressing, whisk all the ingredients together in a bowl. Pour the dressing over the salad and mix gently to combine.

5 Chill the salad, covered, for 1–2 hours to allow the flavors to develop. Check the seasoning before serving and garnish with mint sprigs.

ANOTHER IDEA
+ *For a quicker version, use a can of drained and flaked tuna. Simply toss the tuna with the vegetables, herbs and cooked bulgur.*

Each serving provides
328 calories, 21 g protein, 11 g fat (2 g saturated fat), 31 g carbohydrate (5 g sugars), 8 g fiber, 276 mg sodium

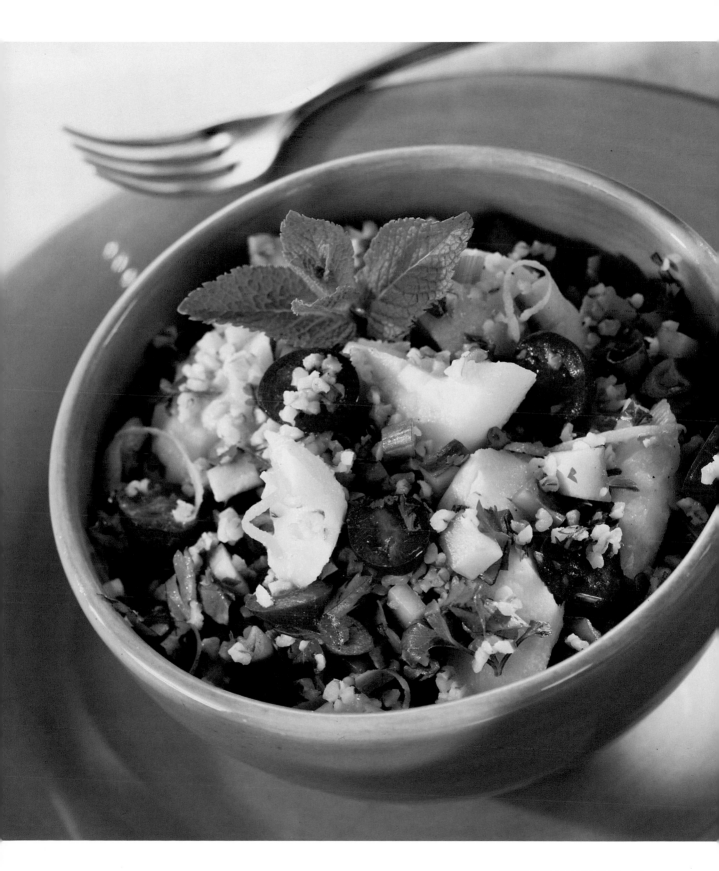

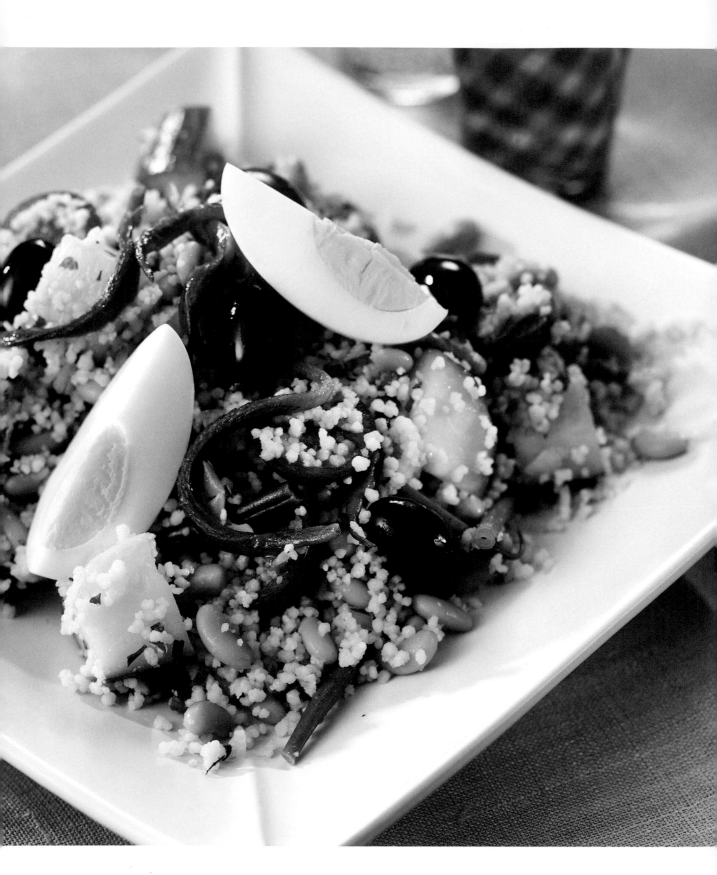

couscous & *cannellini niçoise*

This recipe takes its inspiration from the classic French salad, but with a few twists on the original. Here, couscous is mixed with cannellini beans, and tossed with green beans, tomatoes and cucumber in a piquant dressing made with sun-dried tomatoes.

SERVES 4 PREPARATION 25 MINUTES COOKING 5 MINUTES

1$^{1}/_{3}$ cups (245 g) couscous

1$^{2}/_{3}$ cups (400 ml) boiling water

1 tablespoon (30 ml) extra virgin olive oil

1 teaspoon (5 ml) dried herbes de Provence

$^{2}/_{3}$ cup (150 g) green beans

$^{1}/_{2}$ cucumber

15 ounce (425 ml) can low-salt cannellini beans, drained, rinsed

1 small red onion, finely chopped

1 cup (250 g) cherry tomatoes, halved

2 hard-boiled eggs, cut into quarters

4 anchovy fillets, drained and halved lengthwise

$^{1}/_{4}$ cup (50 g) black olives

Sun-dried tomato dressing

juice of 1 large lemon

2 tablespoons (30 ml) extra virgin olive oil

1 tablespoon (15 ml) finely chopped sun-dried tomatoes packed in oil

freshly ground black pepper

1 To make the sun-dried tomato dressing, combine the lemon juice, oil and sun-dried tomatoes in a screw-top jar. Season to taste with pepper, cover and shake well to mix. Set aside.

2 Put the couscous into a large heatproof bowl and cover with the boiling water. Stir in the oil and dried herbs, cover and let stand for 5 minutes, or until the couscous has absorbed all the water. Uncover, stir to separate the grains and let cool.

3 Meanwhile, steam the green beans for 3–4 minutes, or until tender but still crisp. Drain and refresh under cold running water. Cut in half.

4 Cut the cucumber lengthwise into thick slices, then cut each slice into four wedges. Stir the cucumber into the couscous, together with the cannellini beans, green beans, onion and tomatoes. Add the dressing and toss gently until well mixed. Taste and season with pepper, if necessary.

5 Transfer the salad to a serving bowl. Garnish with the egg quarters, anchovies and olives, and serve.

Each serving provides
349 calories, 13 g protein, 19 g fat (3 g saturated fat), 31 g carbohydrate (4 g sugars), 7 g fiber, 441 mg sodium

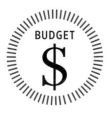
BUDGET
$

COUSCOUS, made from semolina, is the staple food in many North African countries. It is low in fat and needs no cooking.

THE VITAMIN C content in tomatoes is concentrated in the jelly-like substance surrounding the seeds.

ANCHOVIES offer calcium and phosphorus, both essential minerals for the maintenance of healthy bones and teeth.

bulgur, crab & *avocado salad*

Fresh crab is a real summertime treat. It is rich in flavor and works well in this salad with crunchy apples and bean sprouts, chunks of creamy, perfectly ripe avocado and nutty-flavored bulgur.

SERVES 4   PREPARATION 25 MINUTES, PLUS COOLING   COOKING 15 MINUTES

Bulgur salad

1 cup (175 g) bulgur
2 teaspoons (10 ml) extra virgin
   olive oil
3 tablespoons (45 ml) lemon juice
$1/4$ cup (7 g) chopped fresh
   flat-leaf parsley
1 tablespoon (15 ml) snipped
   fresh chives
2 tomatoes, diced
pinch of salt
freshly ground black pepper

Crab salad

$2/3$ pound (350 g) fresh crabmeat
1 avocado
2 green apples
$1^1/3$ cups (120 g) bean sprouts
$1/4$ cup (50 ml) low-fat plain yogurt
1 tablespoon (30 ml) lemon juice
pinch of cayenne pepper
2 baby heads of romaine lettuce,
   separated into leaves
$1/3$ cup (40 g) walnut halves,
   toasted and roughly chopped

1 To make the bulgur salad, put the bulgur into a large saucepan with 5 cups (1.25 liters) cold water. Bring to a boil over high heat, reduce the heat and simmer for 10–15 minutes, or until the grains are just tender. Drain in a large sieve, pressing down well to squeeze out all the excess water. Cool.

2 Combine the oil, lemon juice, parsley, chives and tomatoes in a large bowl. Add the bulgur, mix thoroughly and season with salt and pepper. Set aside at room temperature.

3 To make the crab salad, pick over and flake the crabmeat, discarding any cartilage fragments. Halve, pit and peel the avocado, chop the flesh and add to the crab. Quarter and core the apples, and thinly slice. Add to the crabmeat, along with the bean sprouts.

4 Put the yogurt, lemon juice and cayenne pepper in a bowl and stir to mix well. Spoon the dressing onto the crab mixture and toss very gently until just combined.

5 Pile the bulgur salad onto a platter and arrange the lettuce leaves on top. Spoon crab salad on top of the lettuce and scatter with the walnuts. Serve immediately.

Each serving provides

502 calories, 26 g protein, 25 g fat (4 g saturated fat),
40 g carbohydrate (13 g sugars), 11 g fiber, 436 mg sodium

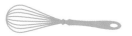

WALNUTS have a high fat content, but this is mostly in the form of polyunsaturated fat rather than saturated fat. Walnuts are a good source of the antioxidant nutrients selenium, zinc, copper and vitamin E.

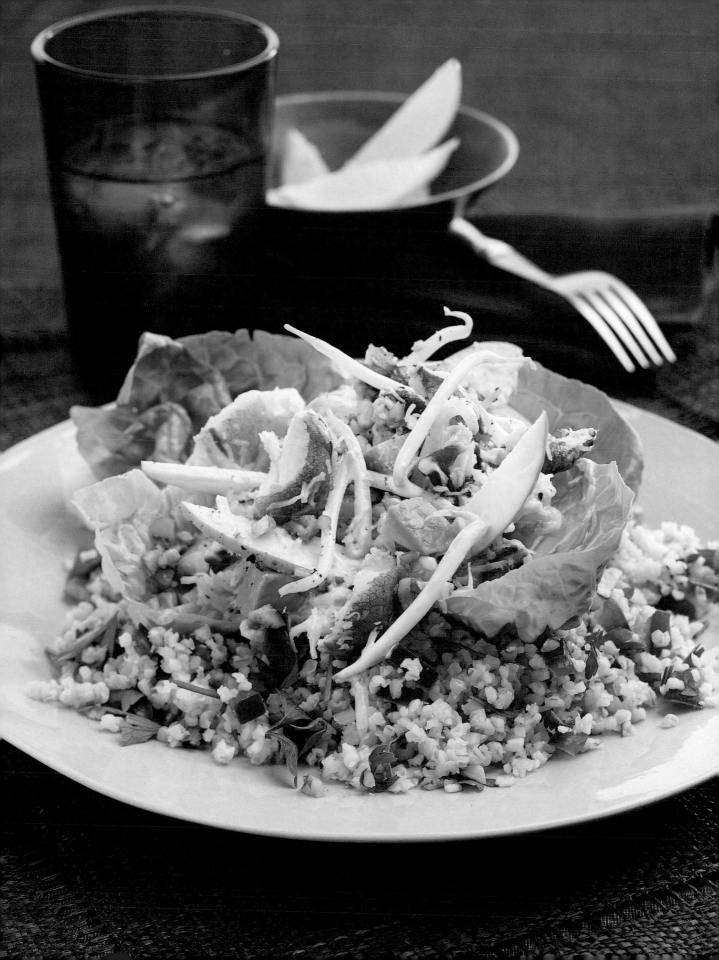

red lentil & vegetable dal

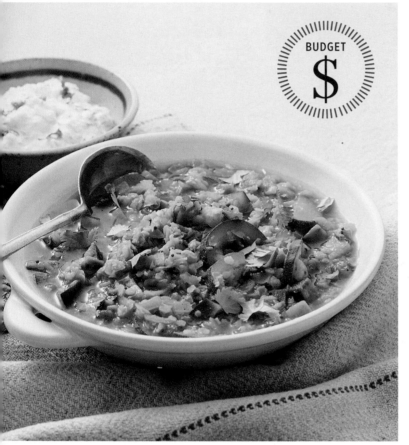

SERVES 4   PREPARATION 15 MINUTES
COOKING 30 MINUTES

1 onion, chopped
2 large cloves garlic, crushed
1 green chile, seeded and chopped
1 carrot, grated
1 eggplant, chopped
1 tablespoon (15 ml) vegetable oil
1 teaspoon (5 ml) ground cumin
1 teaspoon (5 ml) mild curry powder
2 teaspoons (10 ml) black mustard seeds
1 cup (250 g) split red lentils
$1^2/_3$ cups (400 ml) homemade or
   low-sodium vegetable stock, hot
1 zucchini, halved and sliced
1 large tomato, chopped
2 tablespoons (30 ml) fresh cilantro leaves

1 Put the onion, garlic, chile, carrot and
eggplant in an ovenproof casserole dish
or large saucepan. Stir in the oil and
2 tablespoons (30 ml) water. Heat until it
starts to sizzle, cover and cook gently for
about 5 minutes, or until softened.
2 Stir in the spices and cook for 1 minute,
and stir in the lentils, stock and $2^1/_2$ cups
(625 ml) water. Bring to a boil, then add
the zucchini and tomato.
3 Cover and simmer gently for 15 minutes,
remove the lid and cook for another
5 minutes, when the lentils should have
burst open and thickened the liquid.
Serve garnished with cilantro.

Each serving provides
257 calories, 18 g protein, 7 g fat
(1 g saturated fat), 32 g carbohydrate
(8 g sugars), 12 g fiber, 430 mg sodium

DAL is a dish of simmered lentils flavored with
aromatic spices. For an easy low-fat vegetarian
meal, add extra vegetables. Serve with a
selection of Indian-style breads and plain
yogurt or raita.

LENTILS, like other legumes, provide fiber,
and are also a good source of vitamins B_1 and
niacin, both essential for helping the release
of energy from food.

BUDGET $

green lentils with
peaches & red currants

SERVES 4   PREPARATION 10 MINUTES
COOKING 25 MINUTES

1 cup (200 g) French-style
    green (puy) lentils
1 bay leaf
strip of orange or lemon zest
1 tablespoon (15 ml) raspberry
    vinegar
$2/3$ cup (150 g) red currants
1 teaspoon (5 ml) honey
1 tablespoon (15 ml) sunflower oil
2 teaspoons (10 ml) hazelnut oil
pinch of salt
freshly ground black pepper
3 firm, ripe peaches, halved, pitted
    and thickly sliced
1 cup (200 g) mixed salad leaves

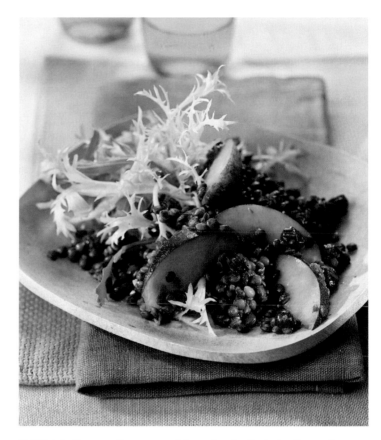

1 Put the lentils in a saucepan with the bay leaf and strip of citrus zest. Cover the lentils with plenty of cold water. Bring to a boil, reduce heat and simmer gently for 15–20 minutes, until the lentils are tender but still firm to the bite. Drain thoroughly and discard the bay leaf and citrus zest. Transfer the lentils to a large mixing bowl.

2 Combine the vinegar, red currants and honey in a small saucepan and add 3 tablespoons (45 ml) water. Bring to a boil and cook for a few seconds; remove from the heat. Scoop out the red currants with a slotted spoon and add to the bowl with the lentils.

3 Whisk the sunflower and hazelnut oils into the red currant juices in the saucepan, and season with salt and pepper. Drizzle the dressing over the lentils and red currants.

4 Add the peaches to the bowl, toss together very gently, taking care not to break up the currants and peaches.

5 Arrange the salad leaves on a serving plate. Top with the peach and lentil salad and serve at room temperature.

Each serving provides
234 calories, 14 g protein, 8 g fat (1 g saturated fat),
33 g carbohydrate (12 g sugars), 10 g fiber, 91 mg sodium

sweet & spicy chickpeas

This colorful dish makes a great vegetarian meal—it's not only healthy but quick to prepare. Like other legumes, chickpeas are an important source of protein for anyone following a vegetarian diet.

SERVES **2**

SERVES 2   PREPARATION 10 MINUTES   COOKING 10 MINUTES

15 ounce (425 ml) can chickpeas, drained and rinsed
finely grated zest and juice of 1 lime
1 teaspoon (5 ml) superfine sugar
1 teaspoon (5 ml) garam masala
1/2 teaspoon (2 ml) ground cinnamon
1 teaspoon (5 ml) dried oregano
2 tablespoons (30 ml) vegetable oil
2 small onions, halved and thickly sliced
1 red pepper, seeded and thickly sliced
1 yellow pepper, seeded and thickly sliced
12 red cherry tomatoes, halved
tortillas, sour cream and lime wedges, to serve (optional)

1 Combine the chickpeas, lime zest and juice, sugar, garam masala, cinnamon and oregano in a bowl. Stir to coat the chickpeas in the spicy mixture. Set aside while preparing the rest of the dish.
2 Heat the oil in a large frying pan or wok over medium heat, add the onions and stir-fry for 4 minutes, or until just beginning to color. Reduce the heat and add the peppers. Cook for another 3–4 minutes, stirring occasionally, until the vegetables are almost tender.
3 Stir in the tomatoes, and add the chickpea mixture. Cook for 2 minutes, or until the vegetables are tender and everything is hot.
4 Transfer the chickpeas and vegetable mixture to a large bowl. If you like, serve with tortillas, sour cream and a squeeze of lime juice.

Each serving provides
341 calories, 10 g protein, 21 g fat (3 g saturated fat), 28 g carbohydrate (10 g sugars), 9 g fiber, 315 mg sodium

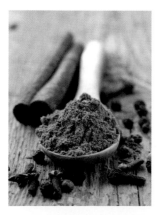

Food Fact
GARAM MASALA, which translates to "hot spice mix," adds a distinctive flavor and aroma to Indian cooking. The main components vary, but it usually contains coriander, cumin, cardamom, cinnamon, cloves and pepper. Garam masala can be used as a flavor base in many dishes, but it is usually added as a seasoning at the end of cooking.

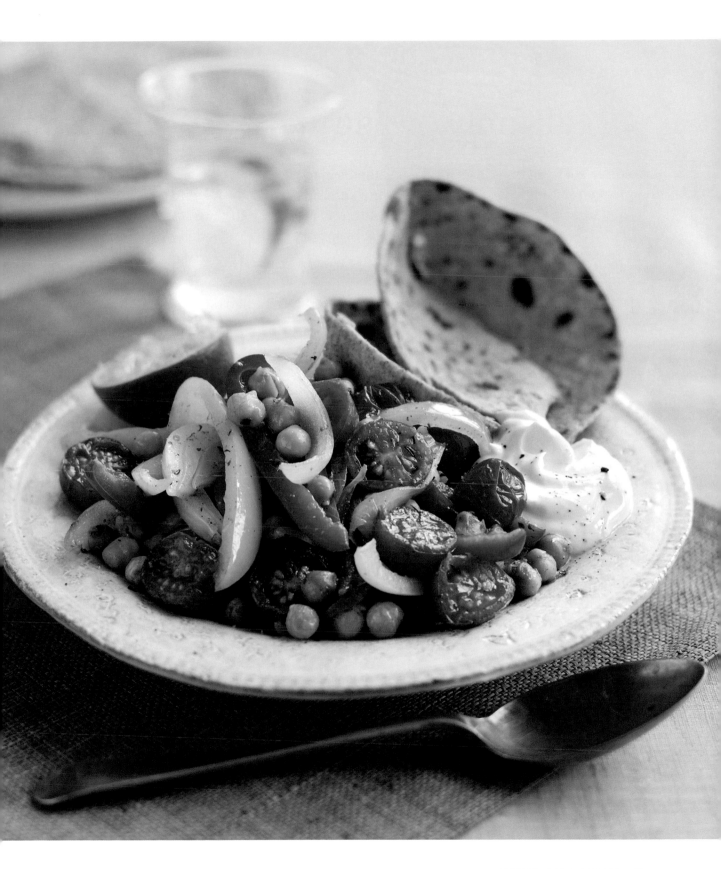

corn & two-bean chili

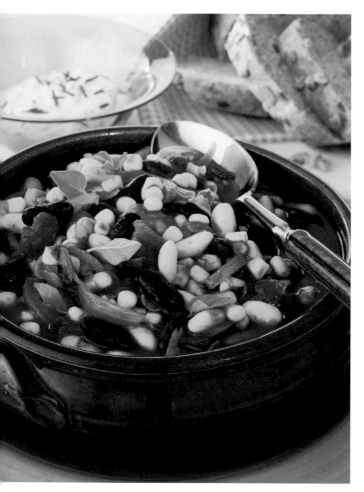

SERVES 4   PREPARATION 10 MINUTES
COOKING 25 MINUTES

2 tablespoons (30 ml) extra virgin olive oil
1 large onion, halved and sliced
1 red chile, seeded and chopped
14$^1/_2$ ounce (400 ml) can no-salt diced tomatoes
2 teaspoons (10 ml) chili powder
1 tablespoon (15 ml) tomato ketchup
1$^1/_4$ cups (300 ml) vegetable stock, hot
1 tablespoon (15 ml) chopped fresh
   flat-leaf parsley
1 tablespoon (15 ml) chopped fresh oregano
freshly ground black pepper, to taste
15 ounce (425 ml) can no-salt red kidney
   beans, drained and rinsed
15 ounce (425 ml) can low-sodium cannellini
   beans, drained and rinsed
1 cup (200 g) frozen corn
1 cup (250 g) fromage frais or
   plain yogurt, to serve
2 tablespoons (30 ml) snipped fresh chives

1 Heat the oil in a large frying pan over medium
   heat, and add the onion and chile and sauté for
   5 minutes, or until the onion is lightly browned.
2 Stir in the tomatoes, chili powder, ketchup,
   hot stock, 1$^1/_4$ cups (300 ml) water, parsley,
   oregano and pepper. Bring to a boil, reduce heat
   and simmer for 10 minutes, stirring occasionally.
3 Add the kidney beans, cannellini beans and
   corn. Simmer for another 10 minutes.
4 Transfer to a serving dish or bowl, sprinkle some
   extra oregano leaves on top and serve with a
   dollop of fromage frais and chives.

Each serving provides
385 calories, 15 g protein, 15 g fat
(3 g saturated fat), 46 g carbohydrate
(19 g sugars), 11 g fiber, 432 mg sodium

LEGUMES have a lot going for them.
They're an inexpensive source of
protein, a good source of B-vitamins
and, when sprouted, are an excellent
source of vitamin C. In addition, kidney
and cannellini beans provide more than
three times the amount of fiber found
in many vegetables.

cheesy chickpea *enchiladas*

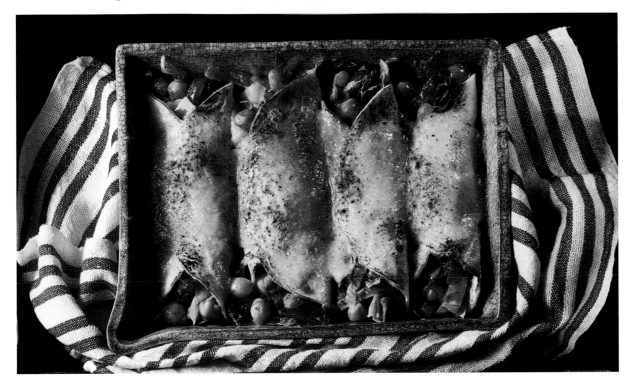

SERVES 4 PREPARATION 15 MINUTES
COOKING 20 MINUTES

2 tablespoons (30 ml) olive oil
1 red onion, thinly sliced
1 teaspoon (5 ml) ground cumin
1 clove garlic, crushed
1 small red chile, seeded and sliced
2 cups (500 g) tomatoes, chopped
15 ounce (425 ml) can low-sodium
   chickpeas, drained and rinsed
freshly ground black pepper
4 large, 8 inch (20 cm), flour tortillas
1 small iceberg lettuce, shredded
1/2 avocado, diced
1/3 cup (60 g) sharp cheddar, grated
low-fat Greek-style yogurt or low-fat
   sour cream, to serve

1 Heat the oil in a frying pan over medium–high heat and cook the onion, stirring occasionally, for 5 minutes, or until softened and lightly browned.
2 Add the cumin and stir to combine, then add the garlic, chile, tomatoes and chickpeas. Cook over medium heat, stirring occasionally, for 5–8 minutes, or until the liquid has almost evaporated and season to taste with the black pepper.
3 Preheat the broiler to high. Place the tortillas on a flat surface and divide the lettuce and avocado among them. Spoon the chickpea mixture down the center of each, fold the sides over, and place in a heatproof dish. Sprinkle with cheese and broil until the cheese melts. Serve with yogurt or sour cream.

Each serving provides
410 calories, 14 g protein, 25 g fat (7 g saturated fat),
33 g carbohydrate (4 g sugars), 7 g fiber, 333 mg sodium

mexican bean burritos

Burritos are a family favorite, and part of their appeal lies in the fact that they are quick and easy to prepare. Once the ingredients are ready, place them in individual bowls on the table, and let everyone assemble their own.

SERVES 4   PREPARATION 15 MINUTES   COOKING 15 MINUTES

2 tablespoons (30 ml) vegetable oil
1 onion, chopped
2 cloves garlic, crushed
1 green pepper, seeded and chopped
1 red pepper, seeded and chopped
1 red chile, seeded and finely
  chopped (optional)
$^1/_2$ teaspoon (2 ml) ground cumin
15 ounce (425 ml) can no-salt red
  kidney beans, drained and rinsed
1 cup (150 g) frozen corn kernels
1 large tomato, chopped
$^1/_4$ cup (60 ml) low-sodium
  tomato sauce
1 tablespoon (15 ml) hot chili sauce
2 tablespoons (30 ml) chopped fresh
  cilantro leaves
4 large flour tortillas
$^1/_2$ iceberg lettuce, shredded
$^1/_4$ cup (50 g) grated cheddar
$^1/_2$ cup (125 g) low-fat plain yogurt

1 To make the filling, heat the oil in a large nonstick frying pan over medium heat. Add the onion, garlic and peppers and cook for 5 minutes, or until the onion has softened. Add the chile, if using, and the cumin and stir for 1 minute, or until well combined.

2 Put the kidney beans on a plate and lightly crush with a fork, then add to the frying pan, along with the corn and tomato. Stir in the tomato sauce, chili sauce and 2 tablespoons (30 ml) water and cook for another 4 minutes. Stir in the cilantro.

3 Meanwhile, heat the tortillas in the oven or in a microwave according to the package instructions.

4 Serve the bean mixture, lettuce, cheese and yogurt in separate bowls for everyone to help themselves. To assemble a burrito, place some lettuce in the middle of a tortilla, spoon some of the bean mixture on top, add some cheese and top with a dollop of yogurt. Roll up and eat immediately.

Each serving provides
404 calories, 17 g protein, 15 g fat (3 g saturated fat),
47 g carbohydrate (12 g sugars), 10 g fiber, 452 mg sodium

FIBER FACT This recipe is high in fiber thanks to the kidney beans, corn and other vegetables. You can increase the fiber content even more by using whole-grain tortillas.

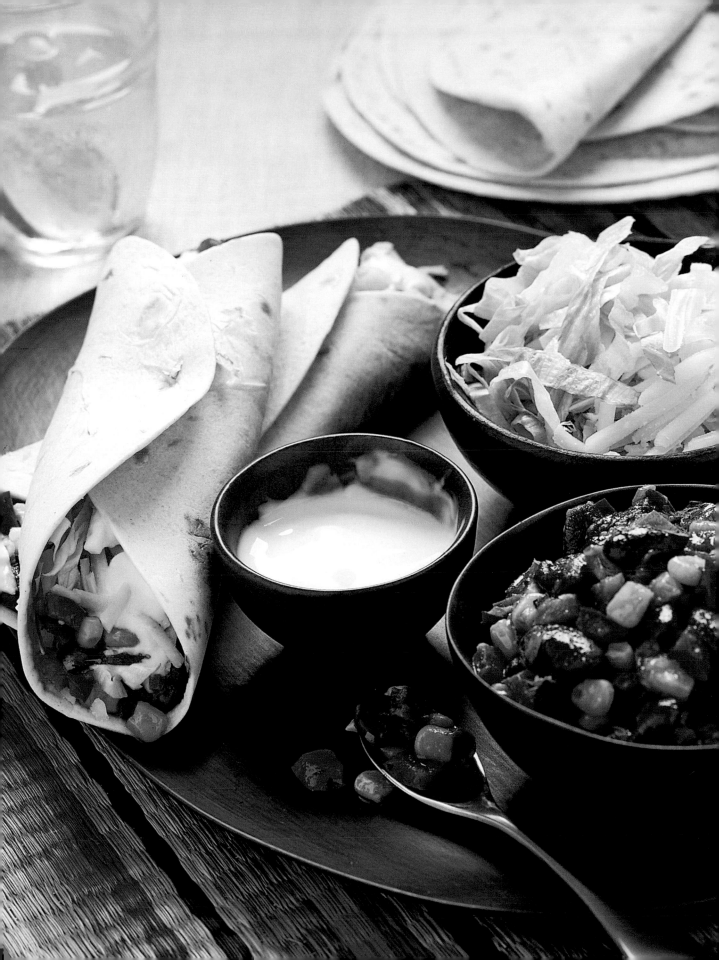

bean tortilla baskets

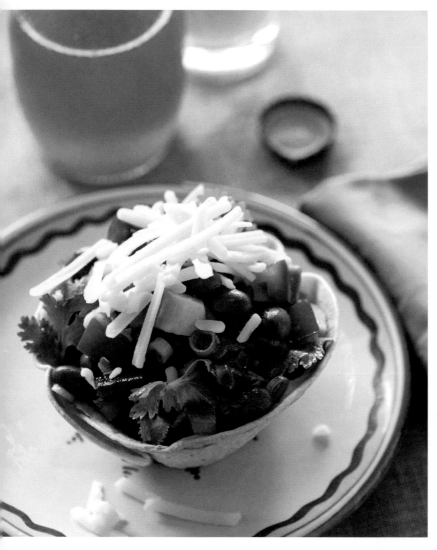

SERVES 2 PREPARATION 10 MINUTES
COOKING 10 MINUTES

2 medium flour tortillas
olive oil spray
1 cup (250 g) no-salt canned red
   kidney beans, drained and rinsed
1/2 avocado, diced
1/2 tomato, diced
2 tablespoons (30 ml) chopped
   roasted red pepper
2 tablespoons (30 ml) cilantro leaves
1 scallion, thinly sliced
2 tablespoons (30 ml) lime juice
freshly ground black pepper
2 tablespoons (30 ml) grated
   mozzarella

1 Preheat the oven to 350°F (180°C).
   Microwave each tortilla for
   20 seconds to soften it, then press
   each one into a 1 cup (250 ml)
   ramekin to create a basket shape.
   Spray with olive oil spray and bake
   for 8–10 minutes, or until lightly
   golden. Allow to cool.
2 Combine the kidney beans,
   avocado, tomato, pepper, cilantro,
   scallion and lime juice in a bowl.
   Season with pepper and gently stir
   until combined.
3 Spoon the bean salad into each
   tortilla basket. Sprinkle with the
   cheese and serve.

SERVES
2

Each serving provides
352 calories, 11 g protein, 21 g fat
(5 g saturated fat), 27 g carbohydrate
(3 g sugars), 8 g fiber, 219 mg sodium

chicken wraps

SERVES 4 (MAKES 8)
PREPARATION 10 MINUTES
COOKING 10 MINUTES

8 medium whole-grain tortillas
1/2 teaspoon (2 ml) cayenne pepper
1/2 teaspoon (2 ml) ground cumin
1/2 teaspoon (2 ml) dried oregano
1/4 teaspoon (1 ml) chili powder
1/2 teaspoon (2 ml) paprika
1 pound (500 g) boneless, skinless
   chicken breasts, cut into strips
2 tablespoons (30 ml) olive oil
1 red onion, cut into wedges
1 red pepper, seeded and cut
   into strips

1 Heat the tortillas in the oven or
   microwave according to the
   package instructions.
2 Combine all the spices in a large
   bowl, add the chicken strips and
   toss to coat well.
3 Heat 1 tablespoon (15 ml) of the oil
   in a large nonstick frying pan over
   medium heat. Add the onion
   and pepper and cook, stirring, for
   4 minutes, or until softened.
   Transfer to a plate.
4 Heat the remaining oil in the pan
   over medium–high heat. Add
   the chicken and cook, stirring, for
   4 minutes, or until golden brown.
   Return the pepper and onion to the
   pan, along with 1/3 cup (75 ml) of
   water, and cook for 1 minute.
   Spoon the chicken mixture into the
   warm wraps. Roll up and serve.

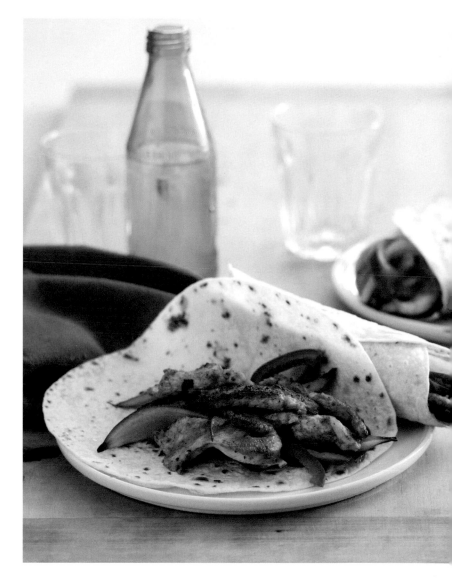

Each serving (2 wraps) provides
420 calories, 33 g protein, 18 g fat
(3 g saturated fat), 33 g carbohydrate
(7 g sugars), 5 g fiber, 426 mg sodium

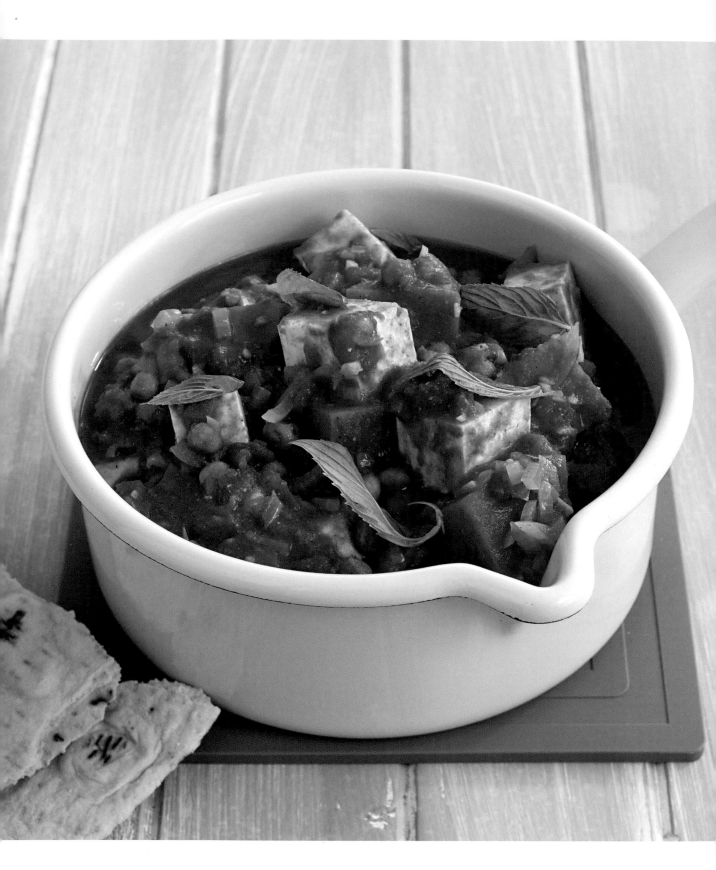

sweet potato curry with paneer

This light, colorful curry is very quick and easy to make and is packed with vegetables rich in antioxidants. Sweet potatoes, in particular, are an excellent source of beta-carotene, vitamin C and vitamin B_6. Serve with naan bread.

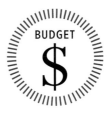

BUDGET

$

SERVES 4   PREPARATION 10 MINUTES   COOKING 30 MINUTES

$1^1/_2$ tablespoons (22 ml) olive oil

1 onion, chopped

2 cloves garlic, crushed

1 pound (500 g) sweet potatoes, peeled and cut into chunks

1 tablespoon (15 ml) mild curry powder

1 tablespoon (15 ml) grated fresh ginger

$14^1/_2$ ounce (400 ml) can diced tomatoes

$^1/_2$ cup (125 ml) homemade or low-sodium vegetable stock

$^2/_3$ cup (150 g) fresh or frozen peas, thawed if necessary

8 ounces (250 g) paneer or firm tofu, cut into $^3/_4$ inch (1.5 cm) cubes

freshly ground black pepper

2 tablespoons (30 ml) fresh mint leaves

1 Heat the oil in a large frying pan over low–medium heat and fry the onion and garlic, stirring occasionally, for 4–5 minutes, or until softened.

2 Add the sweet potatoes and cook, stirring, for another 2 minutes, stir in the curry powder and ginger and cook for 30 seconds.

3 Stir in the tomatoes and the stock. Bring to a boil, reduce the heat to low, cover and cook gently for 12–15 minutes, or until the sweet potato is tender when pierced with a knife.

4 Stir in the peas and simmer for 3 minutes, add the paneer and cook for another 2 minutes, or until heated through. Season to taste with pepper, then transfer to a serving bowl. Scatter with the mint and serve hot.

COOK'S TIP

+ *Paneer is a lightly pressed Indian cheese that is available from Indian grocery stores and larger supermarkets. Firm tofu is a good substitute.*

Each serving provides
328 calories, 14 g protein, 11 g fat (3 g saturated fat), 28 g carbohydrate (13 g sugars), 7 g fiber, 196 mg sodium

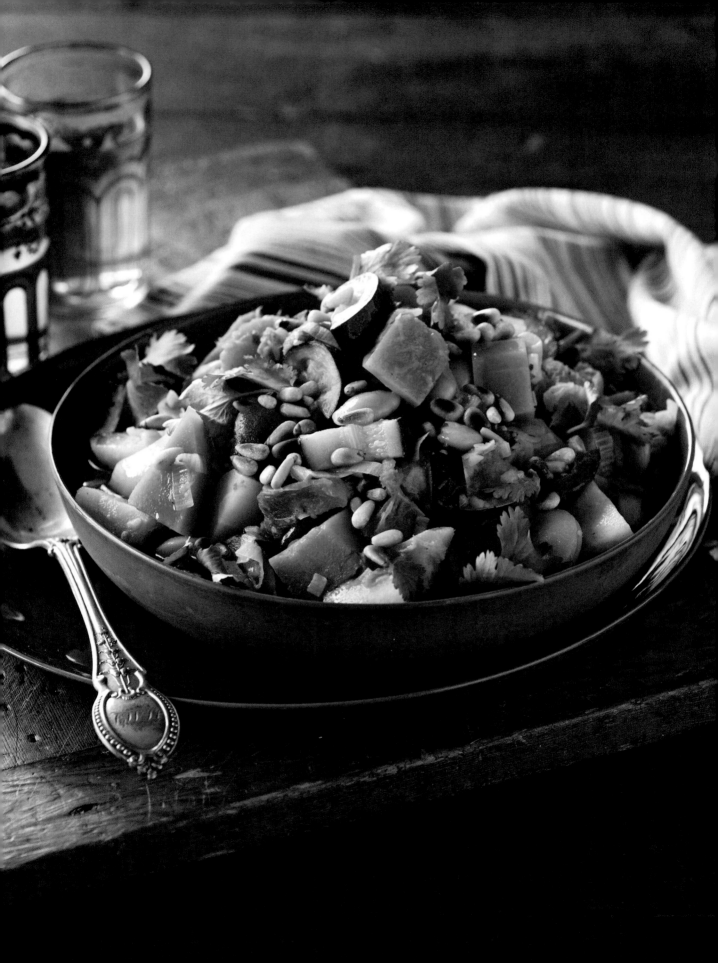

moroccan-style butternut squash & lima beans

Middle Eastern spices flavor this vegetarian casserole, full of vegetables and other fiber-rich ingredients. This is a great recipe for a cook-ahead meal as the flavors will mature and improve when the casserole is chilled overnight. Before serving, remove from the refrigerator and reheat thoroughly.

SERVES 4   PREPARATION 25 MINUTES   COOKING 30 MINUTES

1 tablespoon (15 ml) olive oil
1 red pepper, seeded and chopped
1 leek, halved lengthwise and sliced
15 ounce (425 ml) can can low-
   sodium lima beans, drained, rinsed
1¼ pounds (600 g) butternut
   squash, peeled, seeded and cut
   into 2 inch (5 cm) chunks
2 parsnips, halved lengthwise
   and thickly sliced
2 zucchini, thickly sliced
½ teaspoon (2 ml) ground turmeric
½ teaspoon (2 ml) ground coriander
½ teaspoon (2 ml) ground cumin
pinch of crushed dried red chilies,
   or to taste (optional)
½ cup (90 g) dried apricots,
   roughly chopped
1½–2 cups (375–500 ml) homemade
   or low-sodium vegetable stock
¼ cup (50 g) pine nuts, toasted
fresh parsley or cilantro
   leaves, to serve

1 Heat the oil in a large saucepan. Add the pepper and leek and cook over a medium heat for 5 minutes, or until softened.
2 Add the lima beans, squash, parsnips and zucchini, add the spices and dried chilies, if using, the apricots and 1½ cups (375 ml) of the stock. Cover and bring to a boil, reduce the heat and simmer for 20–25 minutes, or until the vegetables are tender. Check occasionally and add a little more stock if the mixture is too dry.
3 Divide among serving bowls, sprinkle with the pine nuts and parsley and serve.

Each serving provides
301 calories, 10 g protein, 13 g fat (2 g saturated fat), 36 g carbohydrate (21 g sugars), 9 g fiber, 427 mg sodium

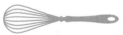

Pine nuts are best toasted as you need them. To do this, spread the nuts in a dry frying pan and cook, stirring, over medium heat for 1–2 minutes, or until they are beginning to brown. Watch them carefully, as they burn easily. Transfer them to a plate to cool.

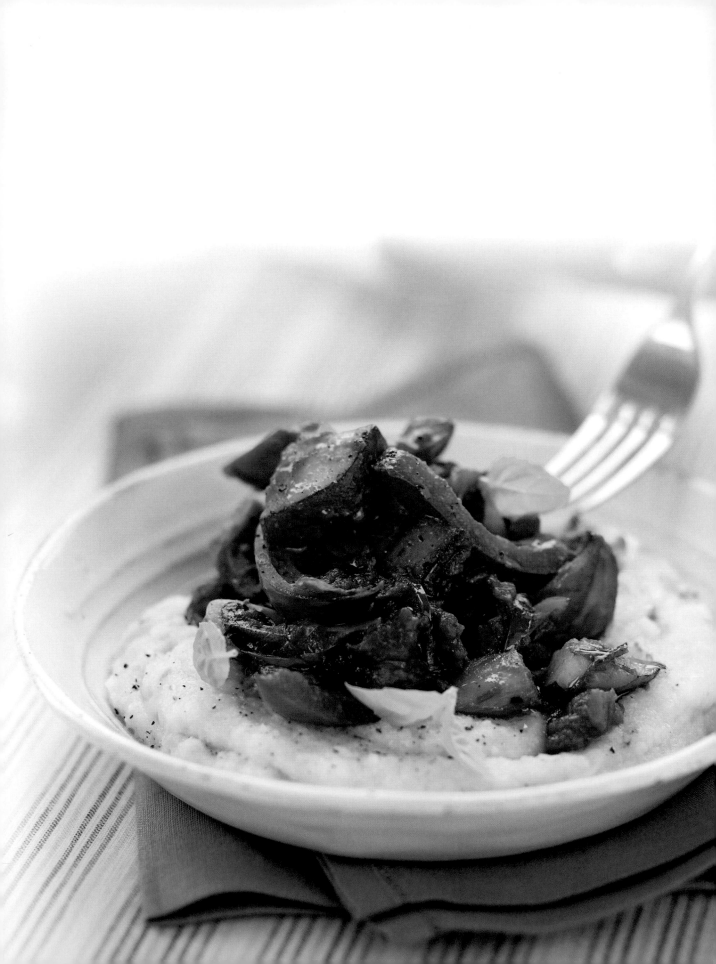

quick ratatouille
with cheese polenta

This dish combines all the wonderful flavors of the Mediterranean. Ratatouille is a traditional French Provençal stew made with tomatoes, peppers, zucchini and eggplant. Here it is served with an Italian-style cheese-enriched polenta.

SERVES 4   PREPARATION 20 MINUTES   COOKING 20 MINUTES

2 tablespoons (30 ml) olive oil
1 red onion, cut into thin wedges
2 cloves garlic, crushed
1 red or yellow pepper, sliced
1 large zucchini, cut into
    small chunks
1 small eggplant, cut into
    small chunks
1 large red chile, seeded and sliced
freshly ground black pepper
14$^{1}/_{2}$ ounce (400 ml) can diced
    tomatoes with basil
$^{1}/_{2}$ cup (15 g) fresh basil leaves,
    torn, plus extra leaves to serve

Polenta
$^{1}/_{4}$ teaspoon (1 ml) salt
1$^{1}/_{4}$ cups (225 g) polenta
$^{1}/_{2}$ cup (125 g) low-fat mozzarella,
    cubed

Each serving provides
393 calories, 16 g protein, 15 g fat
(4 g saturated fat), 48 g carbohydrate
(8 g sugars), 6 g fiber, 367 mg sodium

1 Heat the oil in a large frying pan with a lid. Add the onion, garlic, pepper, zucchini, eggplant and chile, cover and cook over medium heat, stirring occasionally, for 10 minutes, or until the vegetables begin to soften. Season to taste with pepper.

2 Meanwhile, to make the polenta, bring 4 cups (1 liter) water to a boil in a large nonstick saucepan and add the salt. Pour the polenta into the water in a steady stream, stirring constantly with a wooden spoon as you pour it in. Reduce the heat and continue stirring briskly until the polenta begins to thicken and bubble slowly. It should be free from lumps. Half-cover the pan with the lid and cook, stirring often, for 5 minutes. Remove from the heat and stir in the cheese. Season to taste with pepper, cover and set aside.

3 Stir the tomatoes into the ratatouille and cook for another 10 minutes, or until the vegetables are tender. Add the torn basil leaves. Spoon the polenta onto serving plates, top with the ratatouille and serve garnished with extra basil leaves.

ANOTHER IDEA
+ *Make a double quantity of polenta, use half with the ratatouille and pour the remainder into a baking tray, smoothing the top. Cool until set, cover and chill. Cut into wedges or squares. Brush with 2 tablespoons (30 ml) olive oil, and cook under a hot broiler until brown and crisp. Top with a vegetable or meat sauce.*

vegetable &
pearl barley pilaf

SERVES 4   PREPARATION 10 MINUTES   COOKING 30 MINUTES

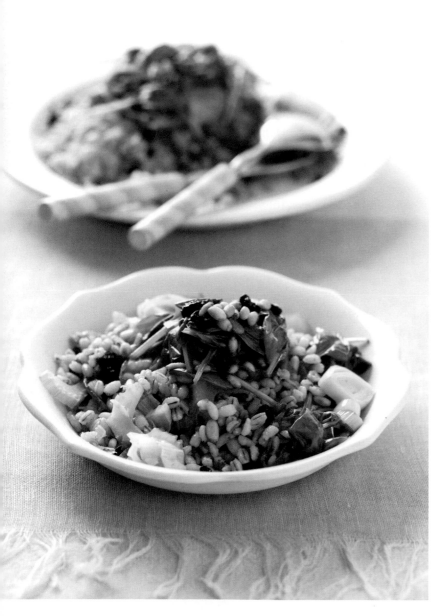

1 cup (200 g) pearl barley
1 bay leaf
2½ cups (600 ml) boiling water
3 tablespoons (45 ml) olive oil
1¼ cups (300 g) leeks, thinly sliced
3 celery stalks, thinly sliced
pinch of salt
freshly ground black pepper
1 cup (250 g) spinach
1 clove garlic, crushed
⅓ cup (50 g) pine nuts
⅓ cup (70 g) dried blueberries

1 Put the pearl barley and bay leaf in a large saucepan and pour in the boiling water. Bring to a boil, stir once, reduce the heat and partially cover the pan. Cook for 25 minutes, or until the barley is tender and the water is absorbed.

2 Meanwhile, heat 2 tablespoons (30 ml) of oil in a frying pan over high heat. Add the leeks and celery and cook, stirring frequently, for about 5 minutes, or until tender. Stir into the cooked barley and season with salt and pepper.

3 Heat the remaining oil in the pan over medium heat, add the spinach and cook for 2 minutes, or until wilted. Add the garlic, pine nuts and dried blueberries and cook for 1 minute. Remove the bay leaf and divide the barley among four bowls. Top with the spinach, blueberries and pine nuts.

Each serving provides
455 calories, 10 g protein, 24 g fat (3 g saturated fat), 50 g carbohydrate (12 g sugars), 13 g fiber, 218 mg sodium

brown rice & *chickpea pilaf*

SERVES 4 PREPARATION 10 MINUTES
COOKING 50 MINUTES

1 tablespoon (15 ml) olive oil
1 large red onion, thinly sliced
5 cloves garlic, thinly sliced
1⅓ cups (350 g) green cabbage,
  sliced
¾ cup (155 g) brown rice
15 ounce (425 ml) can chickpeas,
  drained and rinsed
14½ ounce (400 ml) can
  diced tomatoes
¾ cup (90 g) raisins

1 Heat the oil in a large saucepan
over medium heat, then add
the onion and garlic and cook for
5–7 minutes, or until the onion
has softened. Stir in the cabbage,
cover with a tight-fitting lid and
cook for 5 minutes, or until the
cabbage begins to wilt.

2 Add the rice and 2 cups (500 ml)
water to the pan and bring to the
boil. Reduce the heat to low, cover
and simmer for 25 minutes, or
until the rice has started to soften.

3 Stir the chickpeas, tomatoes and
raisins into the pan; return to a
boil. Reduce heat to low and
simmer for another 10 minutes, or
until the rice is tender. Transfer to
a dish and serve immediately.

Each serving provides
358 calories, 10 g protein, 7 g fat
(1 g saturated fat), 63 g carbohydrate
(24 g sugars), 11 g fiber, 253 mg sodium

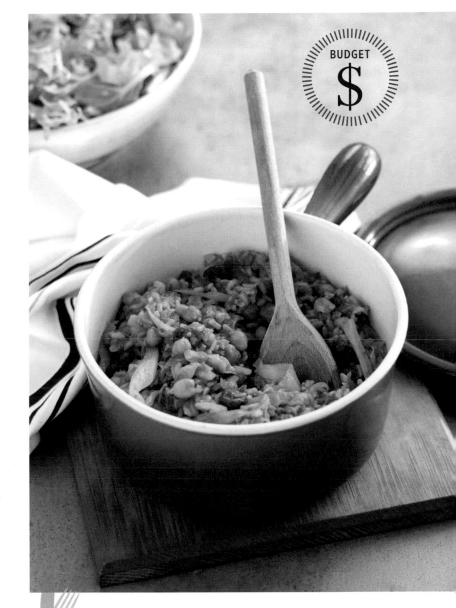

BUDGET
$

FIBER FACT Not only is this pilaf a good source of
carbohydrate, it is also low in fat and high in protein and
a good source of folate. The high fiber content will keep
you satisfied so you won't need a second helping.

potato, corn & *pepper frittata*

Known in Italy as a frittata and in Spain as a tortilla, these flat omelets can be served hot or cold with a salad for either lunch or dinner—and they also make ideal picnic fare.

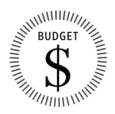

BUDGET
$

SERVES 4   PREPARATION 10 MINUTES   COOKING 15 MINUTES

1^{1}/$_{3}$ pounds (700 g) potatoes, peeled, quartered lengthwise and thinly sliced crosswise

1 red pepper, seeded and chopped

2 tablespoons (30 ml) extra virgin olive oil

1 onion, halved and thinly sliced

1 cup (250 g) frozen corn, thawed

6 eggs

^{1}/$_{3}$ cup (10 g) finely chopped fresh flat-leaf parsley

pinch of salt

freshly ground black pepper

Each serving provides
369 calories, 16 g protein,
18 g fat (4 g saturated fat),
34 g carbohydrate (6 g sugars),
5 g fiber, 260 mg sodium

1 Put the potatoes in a saucepan, cover with boiling water and return to a boil. Reduce the heat to low, add the pepper and simmer for 3 minutes, or until the potatoes are just starting to soften. Drain well, cover and keep hot.

2 Meanwhile, heat a 10 inch (25 cm) nonstick frying pan over high heat. Add the oil to the pan and swirl it around. When the oil is hot, reduce the heat to medium, add the onion and cook, stirring, for 3 minutes, or until soft.

3 Add the potatoes, pepper and corn and cook for another 8 minutes, stirring and turning the vegetables, until the potatoes are tender. Remove from the heat.

4 Put the eggs in a large bowl and beat with a fork to combine. Add the parsley and season with salt and pepper. Using a slotted spoon, remove the vegetables from the pan and add them to the eggs, mixing thoroughly.

5 Return the pan to the stove with any oil that remains from cooking the vegetables. If there are any vegetables stuck on the bottom of the pan, clean and dry it before reheating with 1 tablespoon (15 ml) oil. Heat the pan over medium heat, add the egg mixture, and distribute the vegetables evenly. Cook the frittata, shaking the pan frequently, for 3–4 minutes, or until the edges are set and the top is beginning to look set.

6 Meanwhile, preheat the broiler to high. Place the frittata under the broiler for 2 minutes, or until the eggs are just set—pierce the top with a knife to check that it's cooked.

7 Remove the pan from the broiler and let it sit for 2 minutes, then slide the frittata onto a serving plate. Serve hot or at room temperature, cut into wedges.

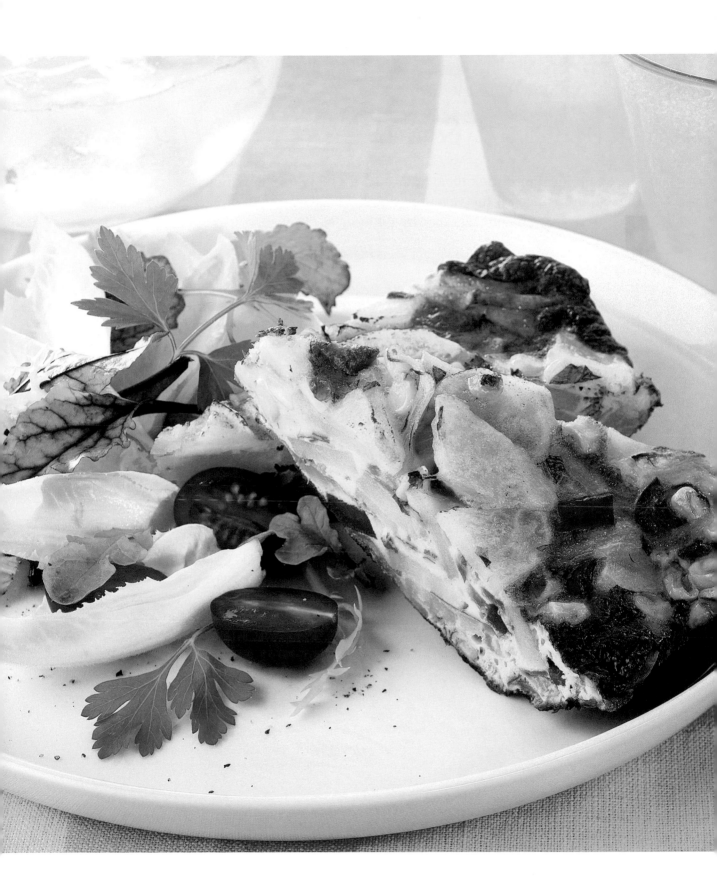

tamarind & *cashew stir-fry*

Here's an ideal midweek meal, packed with tasty and nutritious ingredients. Once all the vegetables and sauce have been prepared, this stir-fry can be put together in a matter of minutes.

SERVES 4   PREPARATION 15 MINUTES   COOKING 15 MINUTES

2 tablespoons (30 ml) sunflower oil
$^1/_3$ cup (50 g) unsalted cashew nuts
1 cup (200 g) sugar snap peas
1 cup (200 g) baby corn, halved
1 red pepper, seeded and cut
　into strips
1 cup (200 g) bok choy, sliced
$1^1/_3$ cups (360 g) fresh egg noodles
1 teaspoon (5 ml) sesame oil
$2^1/_4$ cups (200 g) bean sprouts,
　trimmed
1 onion, thinly sliced
3 teaspoons (15 ml) low-sodium
　soy sauce
2–3 tablespoons (30–45 ml) chopped
　fresh cilantro leaves

Tamarind sauce
2 teaspoons (10 ml) tamarind
　concentrate
1 tablespoon (15 ml) low-sodium
　soy sauce
1 inch (2.5 cm) piece fresh ginger,
　peeled and finely grated
1 teaspoon (5 ml) cornstarch
1 tablespoon (15 ml) dry sherry

1 To make the tamarind sauce, combine the ingredients with 2 tablespoons (30 ml) water in a bowl. Set aside.
2 Heat 1 tablespoon (15 ml) of sunflower oil in a wok or large frying pan and add the cashew nuts. Cook for 1 minute, or until pale golden. Use a slotted spoon to remove the nuts from the wok. Drain on paper towels.
3 Add the sugar snap peas, corn and pepper to the wok and stir-fry over high heat for 2–3 minutes, or until the vegetables begin to soften. Pour in the tamarind sauce, and add the bok choy. Cook, stirring, for about 30 seconds, cover and simmer for 2 minutes. Transfer the vegetables to a warmed dish and keep hot.
4 Cook the egg noodles in a saucepan of boiling water for 3 minutes. Drain, return to the pan and drizzle with the sesame oil. Set aside.
5 Heat the remaining sunflower oil in the wok and add the bean sprouts and onion. Stir-fry for 2 minutes, then add the noodles and cook for 3 minutes, tossing the ingredients together well.
6 Pour the soy sauce over the noodle mixture and transfer to a large serving dish or individual bowls. Pile the warm vegetables on top of the noodles and sprinkle with the cashew nuts and cilantro.

Each serving provides
479 calories, 23 g protein, 18 g fat (2 g saturated fat), 59 g carbohydrate (6 g sugars), 8 g fiber, 445 mg sodium

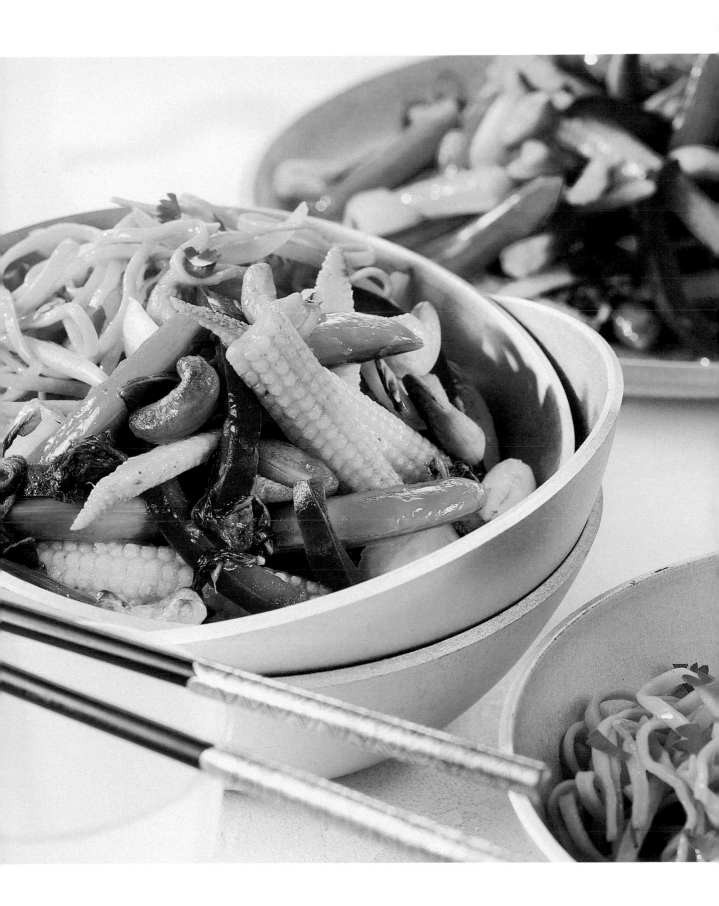

endive & *apple salad*

A light and refreshing accompaniment to grilled poultry or pork, this salad combines crisp apples and sweet dates with slightly bitter Belgian endive and crunchy grated celeriac.

SERVES 4   PREPARATION 20 MINUTES   COOKING NONE

1 tablespoon (15 ml) apple
   cider vinegar
3 tablespoons (45 ml) olive oil
2/3 pound (300 g) celeriac, about
   1/4 large celeriac
2–3 apples, about 2/3 pound (300 g)
1/3 cup (50 g) pistachios
1 cup (175 g) medjool dates
4 heads white Belgian endive

1 Whisk the vinegar and 2 tablespoons (30 ml) of the oil together in a large bowl to make a dressing. Peel and coarsely grate the celeriac, immediately add it to the dressing and mix thoroughly.

2 Cut the apples into quarters, remove the cores, then cut each quarter into two wedges. Cut the wedges in half widthwise and mix with the celeriac.

3 Roughly chop the pistachios. Halve, pit and chop the dates. Stir the nuts and dates into the celeriac mixture.

4 Trim the bottoms from the endives, and separate them into individual leaves, discarding the outer leaves. Arrange the leaves on a serving plate and drizzle with the remaining oil. Pile the salad onto the plate and use the endive leaves to scoop up the salad.

COOK'S TIP

+ *The coarsest disc on a food processor is ideal for grating celeriac. Alternatively, use the coarse blade on a box grater and press firmly to remove good-sized shreds.*

Each serving provides
323 calories, 5 g protein, 22 g fat (3 g saturated fat),
28 g carbohydrate (26 g sugars), 9 g fiber, 38 mg sodium

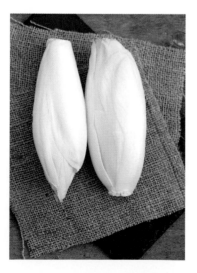

Food Fact
   BELGIAN ENDIVE is a mildly bitter salad leaf, high in fiber, vitamin C and a variety of minerals. The red variety provides good amounts of beneficial antioxidants.

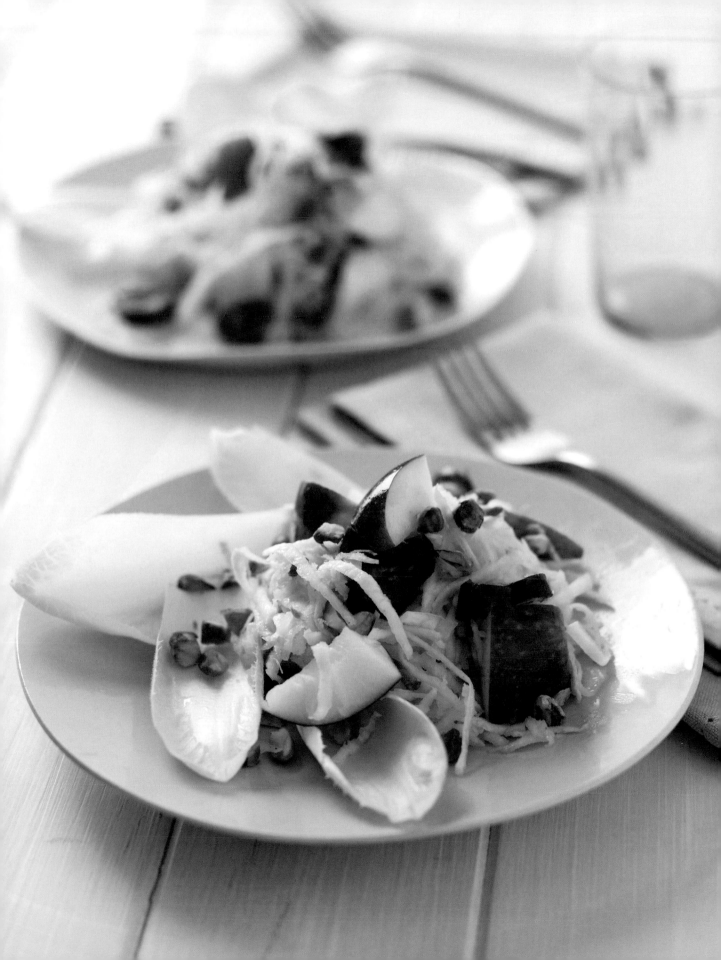

stir-fried beef *with noodles*

Tangy tamarind and fresh lemongrass infuse a Thai-inspired sauce for tender beef strips and rice noodles. With snow peas and baby corn adding color and crunch, as well as an all-important vegetable balance, this is a quick and tasty meal.

SERVES 2   PREPARATION 15 MINUTES, PLUS 10 MINUTES SOAKING   COOKING 10 MINUTES

1/2 teaspoon (2 ml) tamarind paste

2 tablespoons (30 ml) boiling water

2 teaspoons (10 ml) low-sodium soy sauce, plus extra to serve

1 teaspoon (5 ml) sesame oil

2 teaspoons (10 ml) rice wine (sake or mirin) or sherry

1/2 cup (90 g) thin dried rice noodles, such as vermicelli

1 tablespoon (15 ml) sunflower oil

1/2 pound (250 g) lean rump steak, trimmed and cut into strips

1 small onion, cut into wedges

2 teaspoons (10 ml) finely chopped lemongrass

1 red chile, seeded and finely chopped

2 large cloves garlic, crushed

1/2 cup (100 g) snow peas, halved diagonally

6 baby corn, sliced into rounds

1/2 cup (100 g) fresh shiitake or cremini mushrooms, sliced

1 In a small bowl, combine the tamarind paste and boiling water and let soak for 10 minutes, stirring frequently to break down the paste. Combine the resulting tamarind liquid with the soy sauce, sesame oil and rice wine.

2 While the tamarind is soaking, soak the rice noodles in boiling water for 4 minutes, or according to the package instructions. Drain, rinse under cold running water and set aside to drain thoroughly.

3 Heat the sunflower oil in a wok or very large frying pan over high heat, add the beef and stir-fry for about 3 minutes, or until cooked through. Use a slotted spoon to remove the beef from the wok and set it aside.

4 Add the onion, lemongrass, chile and garlic to the wok and stir-fry over a high heat for 1 minute. Add the snow peas, corn and mushrooms and continue stir-frying for another 2 minutes.

5 Return the beef to the wok. Add the tamarind mixture and the noodles and stir for 1 minute to heat through. Serve immediately.

Each serving provides
465 calories, 32 g protein, 17 g fat (3 g saturated fat), 48 g carbohydrate (7 g sugars), 5 g fiber, 447 mg sodium

SERVES
2

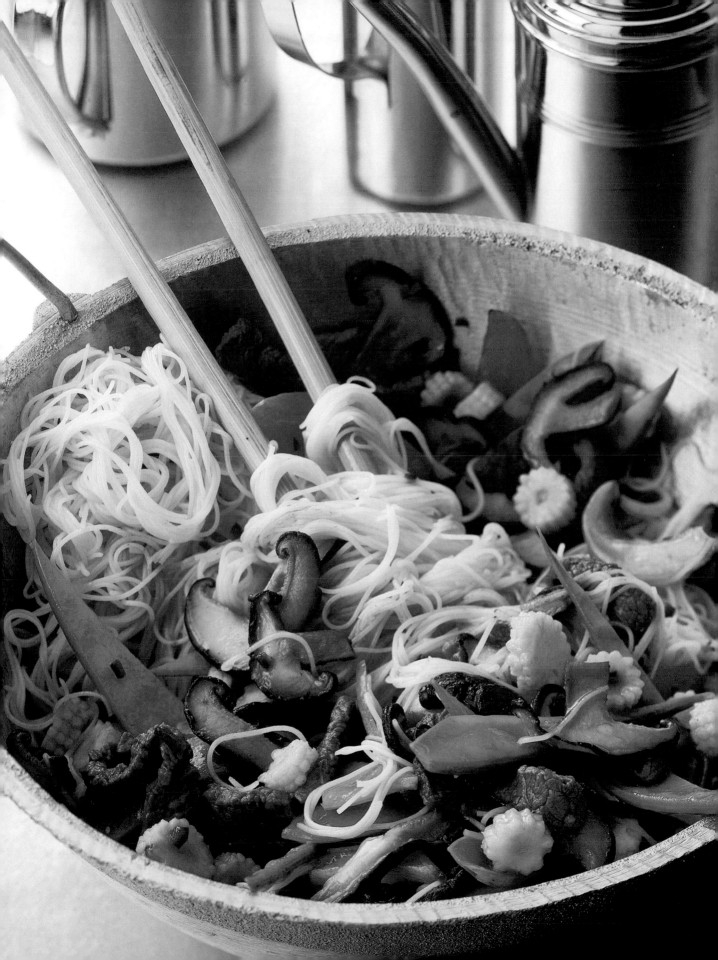

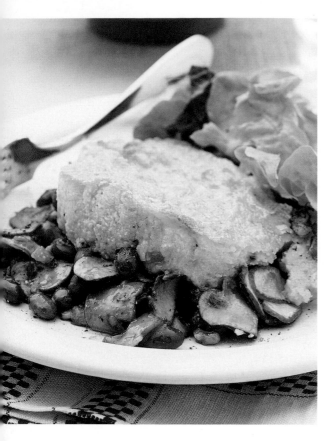

baked polenta with mushrooms

1 Put the dried porcini mushrooms in a small saucepan and add 1 cup (250 ml) of the milk. Bring just to a boil, remove from the heat and set aside to soak.

2 Heat the oil in a wide saucepan over medium heat. Add the celery and cook, stirring occasionally, for 3–4 minutes, or until softened. Increase the heat to medium–high, add the mushrooms and cook, stirring, for about 3 minutes, or until softened. Add the flour and cook, stirring, for 2 minutes. Gradually mix in the remaining milk and cook, stirring well, until the mixture just comes to a boil and thickens.

3 Strain the milk from the porcini and add it to the mushroom and celery sauce. Return to a boil, stirring. Coarsely chop the porcini and add to the pan. Simmer for 2 minutes, add the lemon juice and season to taste with pepper.

4 Pour the mushroom sauce into a shallow ovenproof dish and spread out in an even layer. Scatter the cranberry beans over the top. Set aside.

5 Preheat the oven to 400°F (200°C). Bring 3 cups (750 ml) water to a boil in a heavy-bottom saucepan. Slowly pour the polenta into the boiling water, stirring constantly with a wooden spoon. Reduce the heat and continue stirring until the polenta begins to thicken and bubble. Remove from the heat and briskly stir in the eggs and half of the Parmesan. Season with pepper. Pour the polenta over the mushrooms, and sprinkle the remaining Parmesan over the top. Bake for 20 minutes, or until the sauce is bubbling and the top is lightly browned. Serve hot, with a green salad.

SERVES 4   PREPARATION 30 MINUTES
COOKING 30 MINUTES

1 ounce (25 g) dried porcini
  mushrooms
1²/₃ cups (400 ml) low-fat milk
2 tablespoons (30 ml) olive oil
2 celery stalks, thinly sliced
2²/₃ cups (250 g) sliced cremini
  or baby portabella mushrooms
3 tablespoons (45 ml) all-purpose flour
squeeze of lemon juice
freshly ground black pepper
15 ounce (425 ml) can cranberry
  beans, drained and rinsed
³/₄ cup (170 g) polenta
2 eggs, lightly beaten
¹/₃ cup (35 g) freshly grated Parmesan

Each serving provides
464 calories, 23 g protein, 16 g fat (4 g saturated fat),
57 g carbohydrate (10 g sugars), 8 g fiber, 435 mg sodium

lobster salad *with lime dressing*

SERVES 4   PREPARATION 45 MINUTES
COOKING 15 MINUTES

1 pound (500 g) small new potatoes,
  scrubbed
2 tablespoons (30 ml) low-fat mayonnaise
2 tablespoons (30 ml) Greek-style yogurt
finely grated zest of $1/2$ lime
freshly ground black pepper
1 cooked lobster, to yield about
  $1^2/3$ cups (400 g) meat
2 small shallots, thinly sliced
$2/3$ cup (150 g) snow peas, shredded
$1/2$ cup (100 g) seedless red grapes
$1/2$ cup (100 g) seedless green grapes
$1/2$ cup (100 g) watercress, trimmed
$1/2$ cup (125 g) arugula

1 Put the potatoes in a saucepan and cover
  with boiling water. Cook for 15 minutes,
  or until just tender. Drain and let cool,
  then cut the potatoes in half and place in
  a mixing bowl.
2 While the potatoes are cooling, combine
  the mayonnaise, yogurt and lime zest.
  Season to taste with pepper. Set aside.
3 Pull and twist off the lobster claws and
  set aside. With a sharp knife, cut the
  body in half lengthwise, from the tail to
  the head. Remove the meat from the body
  and tail shell and the claws. Chop all the
  meat into chunks.
4 Add the shallots to the potatoes, along
  with the snow peas, grapes, watercress
  and dressing. Toss to combine.
5 Arrange the arugula on plates and top
  with the watercress and potato salad.
  Scatter the lobster meat on top and serve.

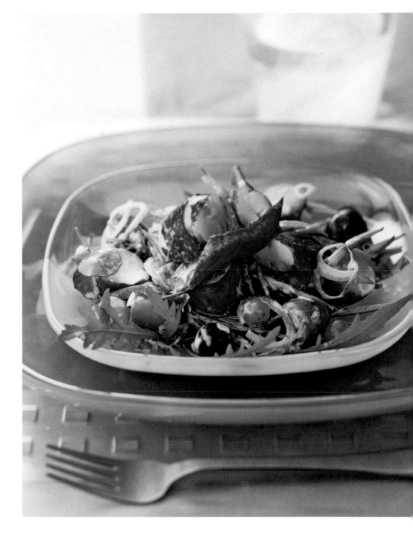

Each serving provides
257 calories, 25 g protein, 3 g fat
(1 g saturated fat), 30 g carbohydrate
(13 g sugars), 5 g fiber, 445 mg sodium

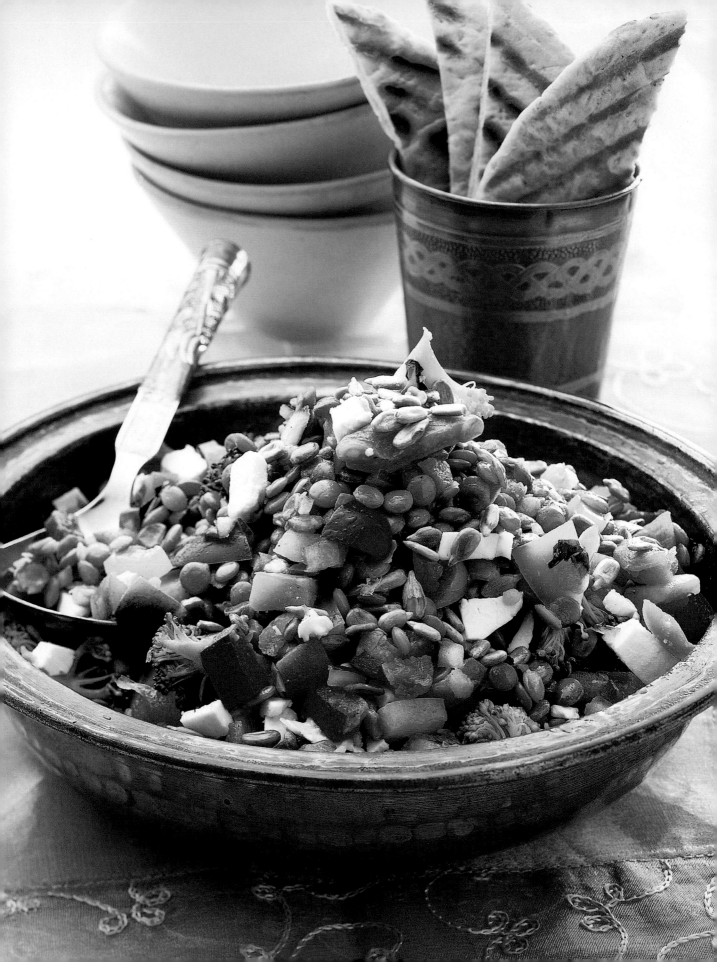

sweet & spicy *lentil salad*

This hearty, satisfying dish is packed with goodness: plenty of fiber from the lentils and apricots and healthy polyunsaturated fat from the sunflower seeds. Legumes contain iron, which is more readily absorbed if you cook or serve them with foods rich in vitamin C, such as peppers and broccoli.

SERVES 4   PREPARATION 20 MINUTES   COOKING 35 MINUTES

$1^{1}/_{3}$ cups (250 g) brown
   lentils, rinsed
1 clove garlic, peeled
good pinch of ground cumin
1 slice of lemon
juice of 1 lemon
3 tablespoons (45 ml) extra
   virgin olive oil
2 tablespoons (30 ml) finely
   chopped fresh cilantro leaves
freshly ground black pepper
1 small red onion, finely chopped
$^{1}/_{2}$ cup (90 g) dried apricots,
   roughly chopped
1 red, 1 yellow and 1 green
   pepper, seeded and cut into
   1 inch (2.5 cm) squares
$^{1}/_{2}$ cup (100 g) broccoli florets
2 ounces (50 g) firm rindless goat
   cheese, roughly diced
2 tablespoons (30 ml) sunflower
   seeds, toasted

1 Put the lentils into a large saucepan, cover with water and bring to a boil, skimming off any scum. Flatten the garlic clove with the side of a knife and add to the lentils, along with the cumin and lemon slice. Reduce the heat and simmer for about 30 minutes, or until the lentils are tender.

2 Meanwhile, to make the dressing, put the lemon juice, oil and cilantro into a large salad bowl, season to taste with pepper, and whisk together.

3 Drain the lentils, discarding the lemon slice and garlic, and add them to the salad bowl. Toss gently to mix with the dressing.

4 Add the onion, apricots, peppers and broccoli to the bowl, and mix gently. Scatter the goat cheese and sunflower seeds over the salad. Serve immediately.

ANOTHER IDEA
+ *Use $^{2}/_{3}$ cup (150 g) frozen fava beans instead of broccoli florets. Cook the beans in boiling water for 5 minutes, or until tender. Drain and refresh under cold water.*

Each serving provides
414 calories, 22 g protein, 21 g fat (4 g saturated fat),
37 g carbohydrate (14 g sugars), 13 g fiber, 78 mg sodium

couscous & *chickpea salad*

This couscous salad is wholesome enough to eat on its own, but it's also a great dish for summer dinner parties because it can be made in advance. Serve with barbecued chicken or fish, or pan-fried lamb chops if you like, and all you'll need to add is a mixed green salad.

SERVES 2   PREPARATION 25 MINUTES   COOKING 10 MINUTES

1/2 cup (95 g) couscous
2 tablespoons (30 ml) currants
3 tablespoons (45 ml) boiling water
2 tablespoons (30 ml) slivered
   almonds
2 tablespoons (30 ml) olive oil
1/2 red onion, chopped
1/2 pepper, seeded and chopped
1 teaspoon (5 ml) ground cumin
1/2 cup (125 g) drained and rinsed
   canned chickpeas
6 pitted green olives, quartered
1 1/2 tablespoons (22 ml) chopped
   fresh parsley
1 tablespoon (15 ml) lemon juice
freshly ground black pepper

SERVES
2

1 Put the couscous and currants in a large heatproof bowl. Add the boiling water and stir to combine, cover with foil and set aside to soak for 5 minutes, or until all the water has been absorbed. Fluff the couscous with a fork to break up any lumps.
2 Meanwhile, toast the almonds in a nonstick frying pan over a medium heat for 3–4 minutes, or until lightly golden, stirring occasionally. Remove from the pan.
3 Heat 2 teaspoons (10 ml) of the oil in the pan over medium heat. Add the onion and pepper and cook, stirring, for 3–4 minutes, or until softened.
4 Add the almonds, cumin, chickpeas, olives, parsley, lemon juice and remaining oil and stir to combine. Add the chickpea mixture to the couscous in the bowl, season to taste with pepper and stir well. Serve immediately, or cover and refrigerate until required.

ANOTHER IDEA

+ *Use any leftover chickpeas to make hummus. Blend them with crushed garlic, olive oil, tahini (sesame seed paste), ground cumin and lemon juice. Spread on sandwiches or use as a dip.*

Each serving provides
459 calories, 12 g protein, 24 g fat (3 g saturated fat),
50 g carbohydrate (4 g sugars), 5 g fiber, 161 mg sodium

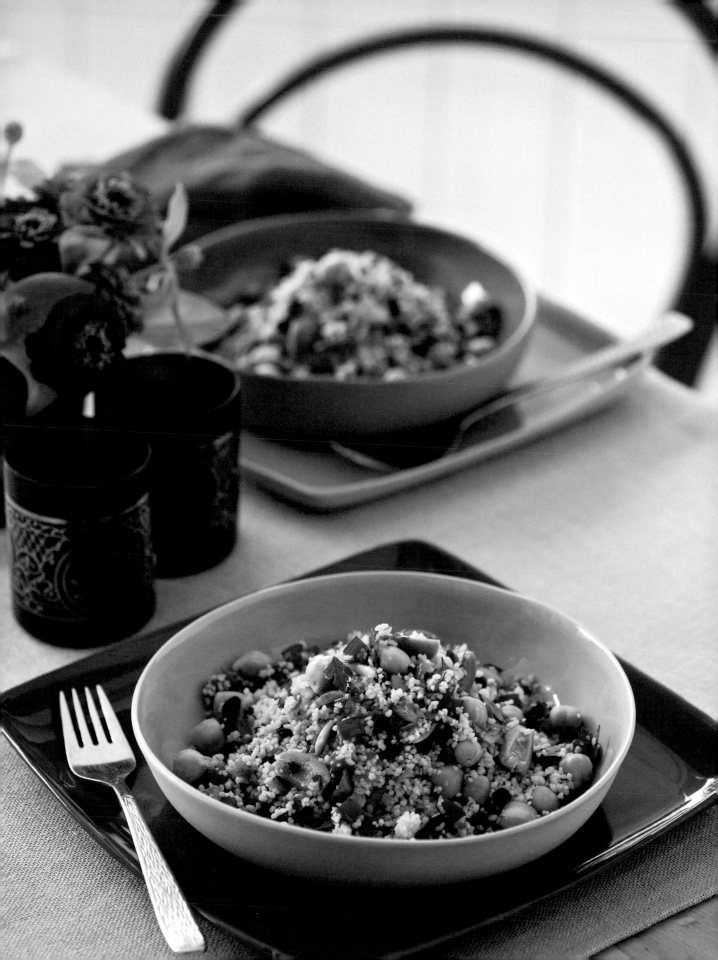

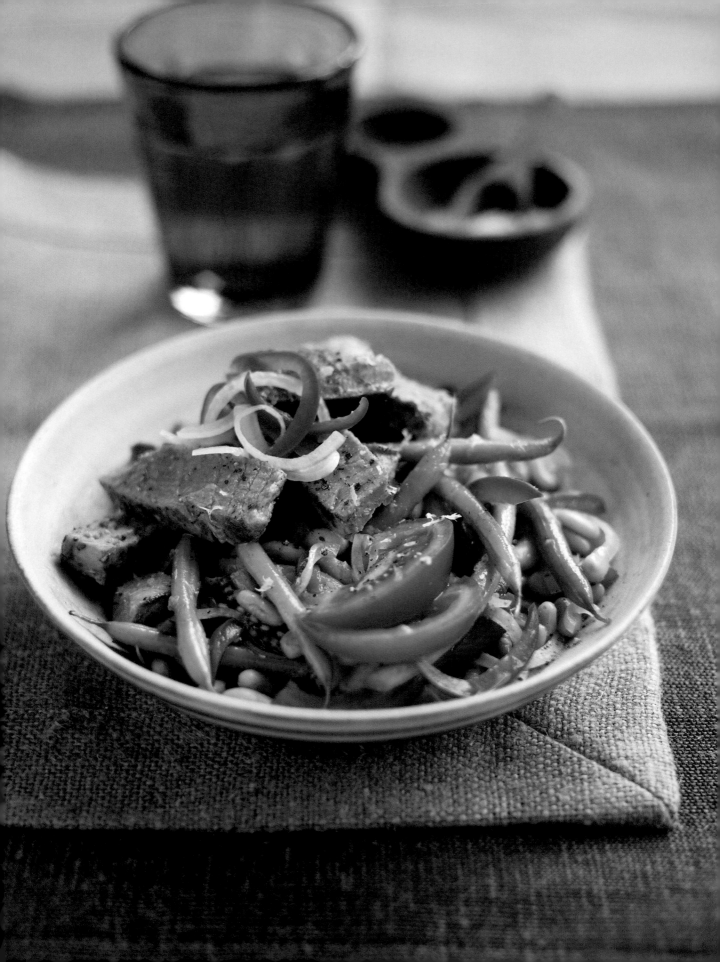

tuna with moroccan spices & bean salad

Ras el hanout, a zesty Moroccan spice mix, is used here to give this tuna and bean dish a punch of flavor. If you like, serve with a watercress and arugula salad and some flatbread.

SERVES 4   PREPARATION 15 MINUTES   COOKING 10 MINUTES

4 tuna steaks, about $1/4$ pound (125 g) each
1 tablespoon (15 ml) ras el hanout spice mix
$1^1/4$ cups (300 g) green beans
2 tablespoons (30 ml) honey
grated zest and juice of 2 lemons
4 tomatoes, halved and cut into wedges
15 ounce (425 ml) can cannellini beans, drained and rinsed
2 tablespoons (30 ml) olive oil
1 small onion, halved and thinly sliced
2 large red peppers, seeded and sliced
2 cloves garlic, thinly sliced

1 Put the tuna steaks on a plate and rub the ras el hanout on both sides to coat. Set aside.

2 Cook the green beans in a saucepan of boiling water for 2–3 minutes, or until just tender. Drain, rinse under cold water, drain again and put into a bowl. Add the honey, lemon zest and lemon juice and mix well. Add the tomatoes and cannellini beans.

3 Heat half of the oil in a frying pan over high heat. Add the onion, peppers and garlic and cook, stirring, for 1 minute, or until very lightly cooked. Add to the tomato and bean mixture and stir to combine.

4 Return the pan to the heat and add the remaining oil. Add the tuna, scraping any spice mix from the plate onto the fish. Cook over high heat for 2 minutes, turn over and cook for another 2–3 minutes, pressing the fish lightly with a spatula, until just cooked through.

5 Divide the bean salad among four plates. Cut the tuna into thick slices and place them on the salad. Scrape any juices and spices from the pan, pour over the tuna and serve.

COOK'S TIP

+ *To make ras el hanout, combine 1 tablespoon (15 ml) ground coriander, $1/2$ teaspoon (2 ml) ground cinnamon, $1/4$ teaspoon (1 ml) ground mace or freshly grated nutmeg and a large pinch of chili powder. Alternatively, use 2–4 teaspoons (10–20 ml) of an African spice paste, such as harissa.*

Each serving provides
391 calories, 34 g protein, 16 g fat (4 g saturated fat), 28 g carbohydrate (20 g sugars), 10 g fiber, 224 mg sodium

MANY PASTA varieties are now available in whole-grain versions. For a higher fiber, healthier lasagna, choose whole-wheat no-boil lasagna sheets (you will need to bake the lasagna for about 10 minutes longer).

lasagna

SERVES 4   PREPARATION 20 MINUTES   COOKING 1¾ HOURS

2½ tablespoons (37 ml) olive oil

1 large onion, finely chopped

4 carrots, finely chopped

2 celery stalks, finely chopped

2 cloves garlic, crushed

⅔ pound (350 g) lean ground beef

⅔ cup (150 g) button
 mushrooms, chopped

⅔ cup (150 ml) homemade or
 low-sodium beef stock

⅔ cup (150 ml) red wine or
 extra beef stock

14½ ounce (400 ml) can no-salt
 diced tomatoes

2 teaspoons (10 ml) no-salt
 tomato paste

1 teaspoon (5 ml) dried oregano
 or mixed herbs

3 tablespoons (45 ml) chopped
 fresh flat-leaf parsley

freshly ground black pepper

10 fresh lasagna pasta sheets

4 tablespoons (60 ml) grated
 low-fat sharp cheddar

White sauce

3 tablespoons (45 ml) cornstarch

2½ cups (600 ml) low-fat milk

pinch of freshly grated nutmeg

1 Heat the oil in a large saucepan over low heat and cook the onion for 5 minutes, stirring occasionally. Add the carrots, celery and garlic and cook, stirring, until the onion is soft and just beginning to color.

2 Increase the heat a little, add the ground beef and cook, stirring and breaking up the meat with a wooden spoon, until browned. Add the mushrooms and cook for another minute. Add the stock, ⅔ cup (150 ml) water, wine, tomatoes, tomato paste and dried herbs and stir together thoroughly. Bring the mixture to a boil, cover and gently simmer over a low heat for 45 minutes, stirring occasionally. Stir in the parsley and season to taste with pepper. Preheat the oven to 350°F (180°C).

3 To make the white sauce, mix the cornstarch and a little of the milk to a smooth paste in a heatproof bowl. Heat the remaining milk to boiling in a saucepan, and pour some of the hot milk into the cornstarch mixture, stirring well. Return this mixture to the milk in the saucepan. Bring to a boil, stirring until the sauce thickens, then simmer for 2 minutes. Stir in the nutmeg and season to taste with pepper.

4 Spoon half the meat sauce on the bottom of a 12 cup (3 liter) ovenproof dish or roasting pan. Cover with half the lasagna sheets, add the remaining meat sauce and cover with another layer of lasagna sheets. Add the white sauce to completely cover the lasagna. Scatter the cheese over the top.

5 Place the dish on a baking tray and bake for 45 minutes, or until the lasagna is bubbling and the top is lightly browned. Remove from the oven and let rest for about 10 minutes before serving.

Each serving provides

610 calories, 38 g protein, 21 g fat (6 g saturated fat),
62 g carbohydrate (19 g sugars), 7 g fiber, 445 mg sodium

herbed eggplant *lasagna*

Fennel, bay leaf, marjoram and sage add flavor to this hearty vegetarian lasagna. The low-fat ricotta topping used here makes this a healthier choice than the full-fat version used in a traditional lasagna. Serve with a green salad.

SERVES 4   PREPARATION 30 MINUTES   COOKING 1¼ HOURS

2 tablespoons (30 ml) olive oil
1 tablespoon (15 ml) fennel seeds
1 bay leaf
1 large onion, chopped
1 clove garlic, crushed
1 celery stalk, diced
1 carrot, diced
1 cup (100 g) chopped mushrooms
3 tablespoons (45 ml) chopped fresh
  marjoram or 1 tablespoon (15 ml)
  dried marjoram
6 fresh sage leaves, shredded,
  or 1 tablespoon (15 ml) dried sage
2 large eggplants, cut into ½ inch
  (1 cm) cubes
finely grated zest of 1 lemon
2 cans, 14½ ounce (400 ml)
  diced tomatoes
freshly ground black pepper
2 cups (500 g) low-fat ricotta
2 tablespoons (30 ml) all-purpose
  flour
1 egg
½ cup (125 ml) low-fat milk
⅛ teaspoon (0.5 ml) freshly
  grated nutmeg
12 fresh lasagna pasta sheets
2 tablespoons (30 ml) freshly
  grated Parmesan

1 Heat the oil in a large saucepan over medium heat. Add the fennel seeds and bay leaf and cook for a few seconds, pressing the seeds with the back of a spoon to release their aroma. Add the onion, garlic, celery, carrot, mushrooms, marjoram and sage. Cook for 10 minutes, stirring frequently, until the vegetables have softened slightly.

2 Add the eggplant and lemon zest to the pan and mix well. Cook for another 5 minutes, pour in the tomatoes and season to taste with pepper. Bring to a boil, reduce heat to low and simmer for 15 minutes. Remove from the heat and set aside; discard the bay leaf.

3 Preheat the oven to 350°F (180°C). Place the ricotta, flour and egg in a food processor or blender and purée until smooth. Add the milk and process again briefly to combine, then add the nutmeg.

4 Pour half the eggplant mixture into a 9 x 13 inch (23 x 33 cm) ovenproof dish. Cover with half of the lasagna sheets in an even layer. Add the remaining eggplant mixture and top with the remaining lasagna sheets, overlapping the pieces neatly. Spoon the ricotta mixture over the lasagna sheets, and sprinkle the Parmesan on top. Bake for 45 minutes, or until the topping is set and deep golden. Remove from the oven. Let stand for 10 minutes before slicing and serving.

Each serving provides
543 calories, 40 g protein, 16 g fat (4 g saturated fat),
60 g carbohydrate (17 g sugars), 14 g fiber, 311 mg sodium

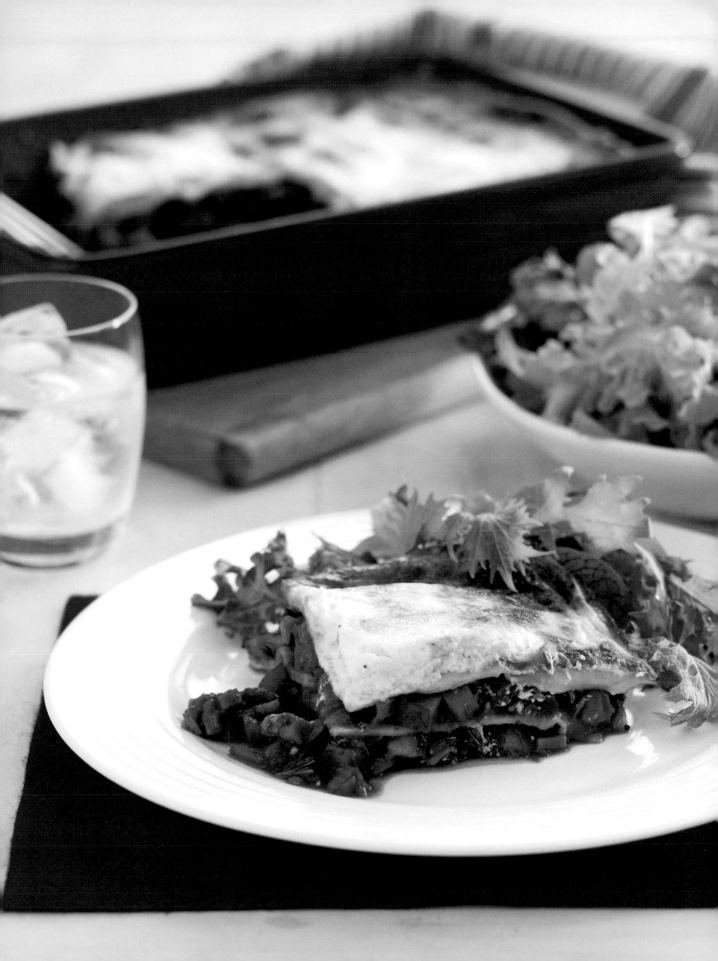

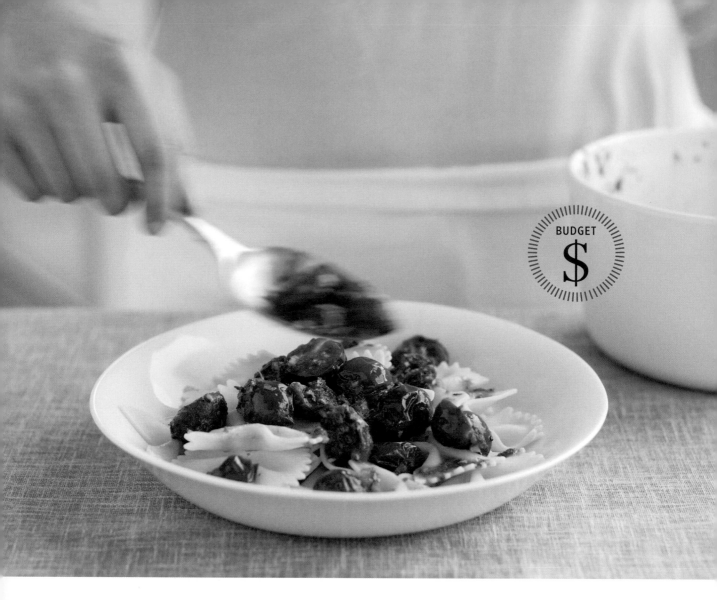

anchovy & cherry tomato pasta

SERVES 4   PREPARATION 5 MINUTES   COOKING 10 MINUTES

12 ounces (350 g) farfalle pasta
1 can, 2 ounces (50 g), anchovy
   fillets, drained
2 cloves garlic, chopped
1 cup (250 g) cherry
   tomatoes, halved
2 tablespoons (30 ml) chopped
   fresh parsley
freshly ground black pepper or
   dried red chile flakes

1 Cook the pasta in a large saucepan of boiling water
   for 10–12 minutes, or until al dente, then drain.
2 Meanwhile, put the anchovies, garlic and tomatoes in
   a nonstick frying pan over a low heat and sauté for
   3–4 minutes, crushing the anchovies a little. Add the
   parsley and season to taste with pepper, then toss with
   the hot pasta.

Each serving provides
312 calories, 12 g protein, 2 g fat (<1 g saturated fat),
61 g carbohydrate (1 g sugars), 4 g fiber, 382 mg sodium

pasta with fresh *tomato & walnuts*

SERVES 2   PREPARATION 5 MINUTES
COOKING 15 MINUTES

6 ounces (160 g) pappardelle pasta
1 tablespoon (15 ml) olive oil
1 cup (250 g) cherry tomatoes,
  halved
1 clove garlic, crushed
$1/3$ cup (40 g) walnuts, toasted
1 tablespoon (15 ml) lemon juice
1 tablespoon (15 ml) finely
  grated Parmesan
10 fresh basil leaves

1 Cook the pasta in a saucepan of
  boiling water for about 10 minutes,
  or until al dente.
2 Meanwhile, heat the oil in a large
  frying pan over high heat. Add
  the tomatoes and cook, stirring
  occasionally, for 2 minutes, or
  until softened and lightly seared
  on the edges. Stir in the garlic
  and walnuts and heat through.
3 Drain the pasta and return to the
  pan, then add the tomato mixture
  and toss to combine.
4 Divide among 2 bowls, drizzle with
  a little lemon juice and sprinkle
  with the Parmesan and basil.

Each serving provides
517 calories, 14 g protein, 25 g fat
(3 g saturated fat), 58 g carbohydrate
(4 g sugars), 6 g fiber, 67 mg sodium

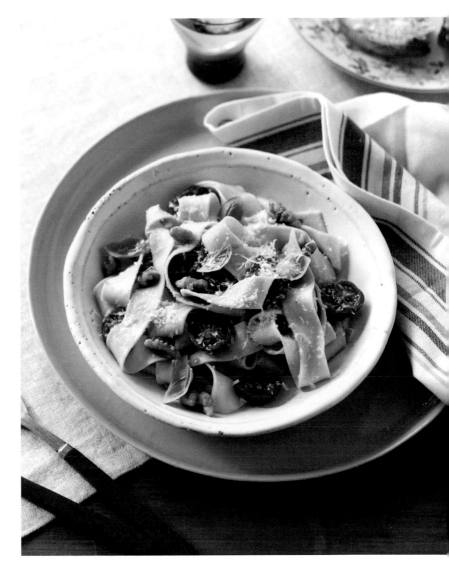

SERVES
2

turkey chili with spaghetti

Sweet peppers and warm spices flavor this chili, which is made with ground turkey for its lower fat content, rather than the traditional beef, and served on whole-grain spaghetti for increased fiber.

SERVES 4   PREPARATION 10 MINUTES   COOKING 25 MINUTES

$^2/_3$ cup (160 ml) low-fat plain yogurt
1 scallion, finely chopped
4 tablespoons (60 ml) finely chopped mixed fresh herbs, such as parsley, cilantro and chives
1 tablespoon (15 ml) canola oil
1 large clove garlic, crushed
1 onion, finely chopped
2 red or green peppers, seeded and finely chopped
$1^1/_2$ teaspoons (7 ml) cayenne pepper, or to taste
2 teaspoons (10 ml) ground cumin
1 teaspoon (5 ml) dried oregano
1 pound (500 g) ground turkey
2 cans, $14^1/_2$ ounce (400 ml), no-salt diced tomatoes
15 ounce (425 ml) can no-salt red kidney beans, drained and rinsed
freshly ground black pepper
8 ounces (240 g) whole-grain spaghetti

1 To make the topping, combine the yogurt with the scallion and herbs. Cover and chill until required.
2 Heat the oil in a large frying pan or saucepan over medium heat. Add the garlic and fry for 30 seconds, then add the onion and peppers and fry, stirring occasionally, for 5 minutes, or until softened.
3 Stir in the cayenne pepper, cumin and oregano and cook, stirring occasionally, for 2 minutes. Add the turkey and cook, stirring occasionally, until browned.
4 Stir in the tomatoes and kidney beans, then season with pepper. Bring to a boil, reduce the heat and simmer for 15 minutes.
5 Meanwhile, cook the spaghetti in a saucepan of boiling water for 10–12 minutes, or until al dente. Drain well.
6 Divide the spaghetti among four plates and spoon some of the turkey chili over each serving. Season with pepper. Serve topped with the herb-flavored yogurt.

Each serving provides
665 calories, 63 g protein, 16 g fat (4 g saturated fat), 63 g carbohydrate (14 g sugars), 14 g fiber, 302 mg sodium

TURKEY is a healthy source of protein. It contains zinc and many B vitamins, particularly thiamin, B_{12} and niacin. Turkey also provides iron and is a good choice because it's very lean.

RED KIDNEY BEANS are low in fat and rich in low-GI carbohydrate. They provide good amounts of thiamin and niacin, and useful amounts of iron. They are also a good source of soluble fiber.

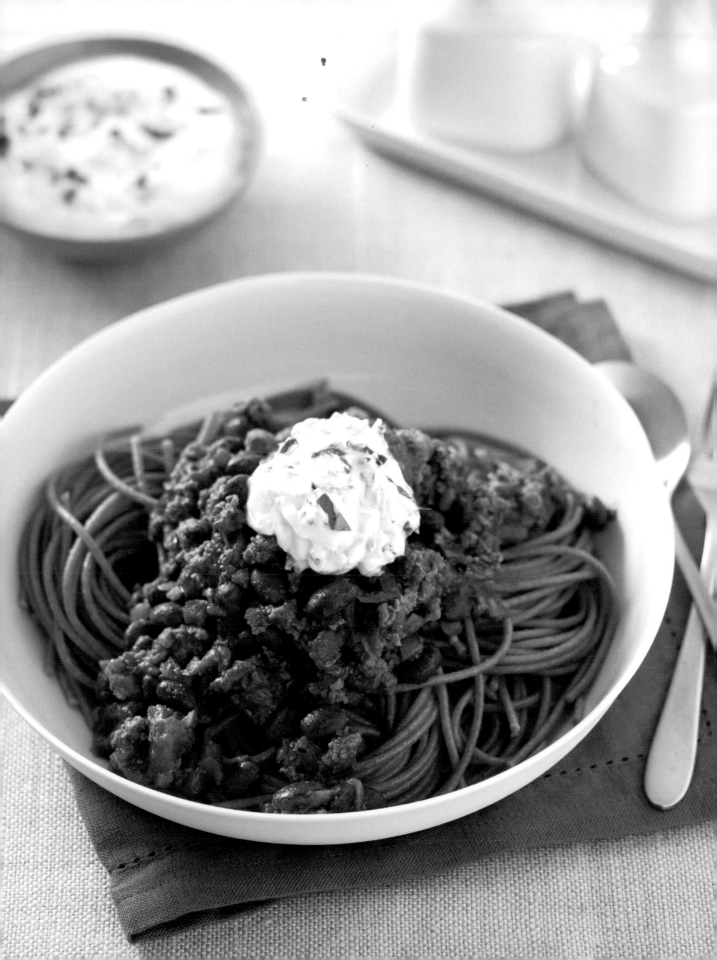

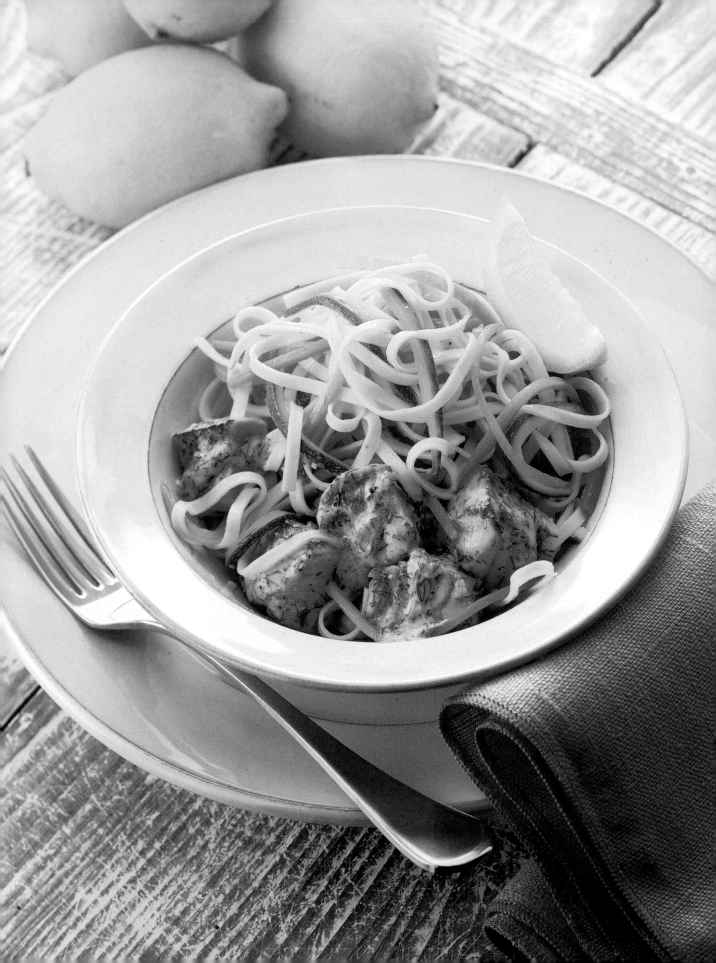

linguine with pan-fried salmon

All the ingredients for this dish are quickly assembled and cooked, making it an ideal weeknight family dinner. The carrots and zucchini are cut into strips and mixed with the linguine—a clever way of including more vegetables in your diet.

SERVES 4   PREPARATION 10 MINUTES, PLUS MARINATING   COOKING 15 MINUTES

3/4 pound (400 g) boneless, skinless salmon fillet
grated zest and juice of 1 lemon
2 tablespoons (30 ml) chopped fresh dill
12 ounces (350 g) linguine
1 cup (250 g) carrots, cut into long matchstick strips
1 cup (250 g) zucchini, cut into long matchstick strips
1 teaspoon (5 ml) sunflower oil
1/3 cup (90 ml) low-fat crème fraîche or low-fat sour cream
pinch of salt
freshly ground black pepper
1 lemon, cut into wedges, to serve

1 Cut the salmon into bite-sized pieces and place in a dish. Combine the lemon zest, juice and dill and add to the salmon. Turn the pieces of salmon to coat them evenly in the marinade. Cover and marinate in the fridge for at least 10 minutes.

2 Cook the pasta in a saucepan of boiling water for about 10 minutes, or until al dente. Add the carrots to the pasta for the final 2 minutes of cooking time, then add the zucchini 1 minute later.

3 Meanwhile, brush a nonstick or heavy-bottom frying pan with the oil and place over medium heat. Drain the salmon, reserving the lemon juice marinade. Add the salmon to the hot pan and cook, turning the pieces occasionally, for 3–4 minutes, or until the fish is firm and just cooked through.

4 Add the reserved marinade and crème fraîche to the salmon and cook for a few seconds. Remove the pan from the heat and season with salt and pepper.

5 Drain the pasta and vegetables and divide among four bowls or plates. Add the salmon mixture and serve with the lemon wedges.

Each serving provides
490 calories, 32 g protein, 10 g fat (2 g saturated fat),
66 g carbohydrate (5 g sugars), 6 g fiber, 230 mg sodium

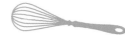

SALMON is an oily fish rich in omega-3 fatty acids, which can help to reduce the risk of heart disease.

whole-grain pasta with broccoli & tuna

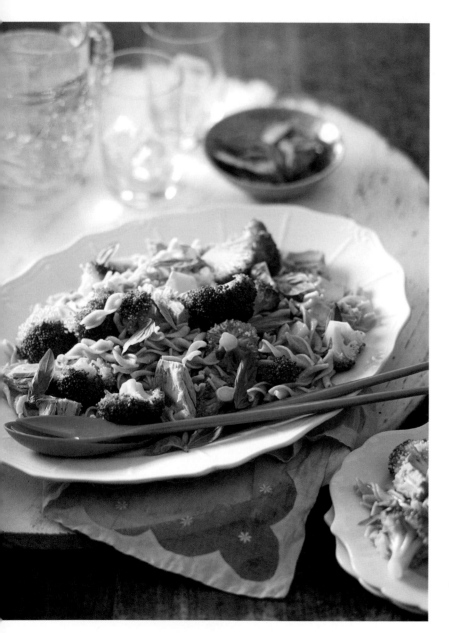

SERVES 4   PREPARATION 10 MINUTES
COOKING 15 MINUTES

10 ounces (300 g) whole-grain
   pasta spirals
1 pound (500 g) broccoli, cut
   into florets
2 tablespoons (30 ml) red
   wine vinegar
$1\frac{1}{2}$ tablespoons (22 ml) extra
   virgin olive oil
15 ounce (425 g) can tuna in olive oil
$\frac{1}{3}$ cup (10 g) fresh basil, torn
freshly ground black pepper
$\frac{1}{2}$ lemon

1 Cook pasta in boiling water for
   10–12 minutes until al dente. Add
   the broccoli for the final 2 minutes
   of cook time. Drain. Return the
   pasta and broccoli to the pan.
2 Meanwhile, put the vinegar and
   extra virgin olive oil in a small
   bowl and stir to combine well.
3 Drain tuna reserving 1 tablespoon
   (15 ml) of oil. Break up the tuna
   with a fork; add the tuna and
   reserved oil to the pan. Add basil,
   and vinegar and oil mixture; gently
   toss to combine. Season with
   pepper and lemon juice, and serve.

Each serving provides
561 calories, 36 g protein, 25 g fat
(4 g saturated fat), 46 g carbohydrate
(1 g sugars), 13 g fiber, 410 mg sodium

hoisin chicken *& noodles*

SERVES 4   PREPARATION 10 MINUTES
COOKING 15 MINUTES

15 ounces (450 g) fresh, flat
  rice noodles
1 pound (500 g) boneless, skinless
  chicken thighs
cooking oil spray
$1^2/_3$ cups (400 g) fresh or frozen
  stir-fry vegetables
$2^1/_2$ tablespoons (37 ml) hoisin sauce
$1/_3$ cup (50 g) cashew nuts, toasted

1 Bring a saucepan of water to a
  boil over high heat. Add noodles
  and cook, stirring, for 3 minutes,
  or until noodles separate. Drain.
2 Meanwhile, cut the chicken into
  1 inch (2.5 cm) cubes. Spray a
  nonstick wok with cooking oil
  spray and heat over high heat.
  Working in two batches, add the
  chicken to the wok and stir-fry for
  about 3 minutes, or until browned
  and cooked. Transfer to a bowl.
3 Add the mixed vegetables and
  2 tablespoons (30 ml) water to the
  wok and stir-fry for 3 minutes, or
  until the vegetables are just tender.
  Return the chicken and its juices
  to the wok, and add the hoisin
  sauce and cashews. Stir-fry for
  2 minutes, or until well combined.
4 Divide the noodles among serving
  bowls. Spoon the chicken and
  vegetables on top and serve.

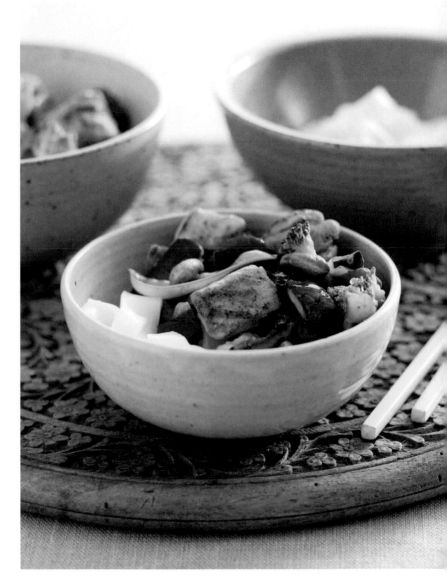

Each serving provides
466 calories, 30 g protein, 21 g fat
(5 g saturated fat), 38 g carbohydrate
(8 g sugars), 6 g fiber, 353 mg sodium

poultry, meat
& seafood

chapter 4

curried chicken & vegetables

SERVES 4   PREPARATION 15 MINUTES
COOKING 35 MINUTES

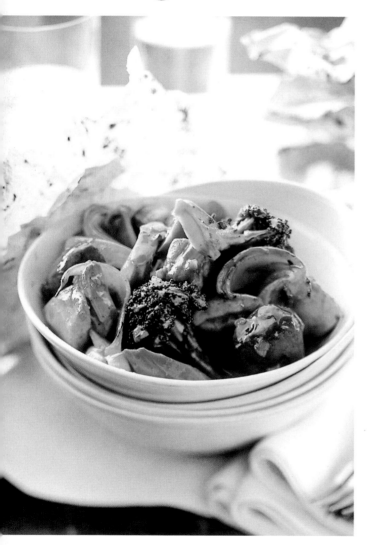

1 tablespoon (15 ml) turmeric
1½ teaspoons (7 ml) ground ginger
½ teaspoon (2 ml) ground cinnamon
½ teaspoon (2 ml) sugar
½ teaspoon (2 ml) freshly ground black pepper
1¼ pounds (600 g) boneless, skinless chicken
   thighs, cut into 1 inch (2.5 cm) pieces
2 teaspoons (10 ml) olive oil
1 onion, thickly sliced
4 cloves garlic, crushed
3 carrots, thickly sliced
1¼ pounds (600 g) small red-skinned
   potatoes, quartered
2 teaspoons (10 ml) creamy peanut butter
4 cups (250 g) small broccoli florets

1 Combine the turmeric, ginger, cinnamon, sugar
  and pepper in a large bowl. Add the chicken
  pieces, tossing well to evenly coat in the spices.
2 Heat the oil in a flameproof casserole dish or
  wok over medium heat. Add the onion and
  garlic and cook for 5 minutes, stirring
  frequently, or until the onion softens.
3 Add the carrots, potatoes and peanut butter
  to the dish with ½ cup (125 ml) water. Bring
  to a boil, reduce heat to medium and simmer
  for 5 minutes, or until carrots begin to soften.
4 Add the chicken and cook for 2 minutes, or
  until it is no longer pink, then stir in 2 cups
  (500 ml) water. Return to a boil, reduce
  the heat to low, cover and simmer for
  15 minutes, or until the chicken is cooked
  through and the potatoes are tender.
5 Just before you are ready to serve, add the
  broccoli and cook for 5 minutes, or until the
  broccoli is tender. Remove from the heat, divide
  among serving bowls and serve immediately.
  Serve with steamed brown or white rice.

Each serving provides
399 calories, 37 g protein, 16 g fat
(4 g saturated fat), 28 g carbohydrate
(5 g sugars), 9 g fiber, 199 mg sodium

thyme chicken with root vegetables

SERVES 4   PREPARATION 15 MINUTES   COOKING 1 HOUR

1²/₃ pounds (800 g) potatoes, cut into
 large chunks
4 baby parsnips, cut into quarters lengthwise
4 carrots, cut in half lengthwise
1 red onion, quartered
3¹/₂ tablespoons (52 ml) olive oil
1 tablespoon (15 ml) honey
1 orange, quartered
4 boneless, skinless chicken breasts,
 ¹/₄ pound (125 g) each
pinch of salt
freshly ground black pepper
a few sprigs fresh thyme or rosemary,
 or ¹/₂ teaspoon (2 ml) dried

1 Preheat the oven to 375°F (190°C). Parboil the
 potatoes for 5 minutes; drain. Return potatoes
 to the pan, cover and shake the pan vigorously
 to roughen the edges (this makes for crispier
 potatoes when they are being roasted).

2 Put the potatoes, parsnips, carrots and onion
 in a large roasting pan. Add oil, honey and juice
 from the orange quarters in a small bowl and
 stir to combine. Drizzle over the vegetables and
 toss to coat evenly. Cut three shallow slashes in
 each chicken breast. Place the chicken among
 the vegetables, along with the squeezed orange
 quarters. Season with the salt and pepper and
 poke in the herb sprigs.

3 Roast the chicken and vegetables, turning the
 vegetables over occasionally, for 50–60 minutes,
 or until the chicken is golden and cooked
 through and all the vegetables are tender.

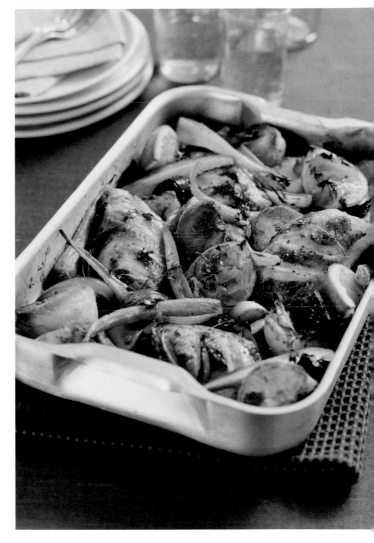

Each serving provides
511 calories, 33 g protein, 23 g fat
(4 g saturated fat), 42 g carbohydrate
(15 g sugars), 7 g fiber, 268 mg sodium

chicken biryani *with raita*

A biryani consists of curried meat, poultry, fish or vegetables combined with basmati rice to make a hearty meal. Here a chicken curry is layered with the rice, baked and served with a fresh cucumber raita.

SERVES 4   PREPARATION 25 MINUTES   COOKING 1½ HOURS

1 tablespoon (15 ml) sunflower oil

1 large onion, chopped

1 pound (500 g) boneless, skinless chicken thighs, cut into 1 inch (2.5 cm) pieces

1 tablespoon (15 ml) chopped ginger

1 small red chile, seeded, chopped

seeds of 10 cardamom pods, crushed

1 tablespoon (15 ml) ground cumin

1 tablespoon (15 ml) ground coriander

6 cloves

1 cinnamon stick

2 bay leaves

½ teaspoon (2 ml) crushed black peppercorns

14½ ounce (400 ml) can diced tomatoes

1 cup (250 ml) chicken stock

½ cup (60 g) raisins

pinch of salt

1 cup (200 g) basmati rice, rinsed

½ teaspoon (2 ml) turmeric

⅓ cup (30 g) slivered almonds, toasted

Cucumber raita

⅓ cup (90 ml) Greek-style yogurt

½ cup (125 ml) low-fat plain yogurt

½ cucumber, grated, squeezed dry

2 tablespoons (30 ml) chopped fresh mint

1 Heat the oil in a large frying pan over medium heat, add the onion and cook for 5 minutes, or until softened. Add the chicken and cook for 5 minutes, or until brown all over. Stir in the ginger, chile, cardamom, cumin, coriander, cloves, cinnamon stick, bay leaves and peppercorns. Cook for 1 minute, stirring constantly so the spices do not burn.

2 Add the tomatoes, stock, 3 tablespoons (45 ml) water, the raisins and salt. Bring to a boil, reduce the heat to low, cover and cook for 45 minutes.

3 Meanwhile, preheat the oven to 325°F (160°C). Put the rice in a saucepan, add 2½ cups (600 ml) water and the turmeric and bring to a boil. Cover and simmer very gently for about 7 minutes, or until the rice is almost tender. Drain excess water.

4 Layer the chicken curry and rice in a casserole dish. Cover and cook in the oven for 25 minutes, checking after 20 minutes and adding a little more water if needed (there should be enough liquid for the rice to complete cooking).

5 Meanwhile, to make the raita, combine the yogurts, cucumber and mint. When the biryani is ready, stir it well, then scatter the toasted almonds on top. Serve with the raita.

Each serving provides
564 calories, 36 g protein, 19 g fat (4 g saturated fat), 65 g carbohydrate (21 g sugars), 5 g fiber, 428 mg sodium

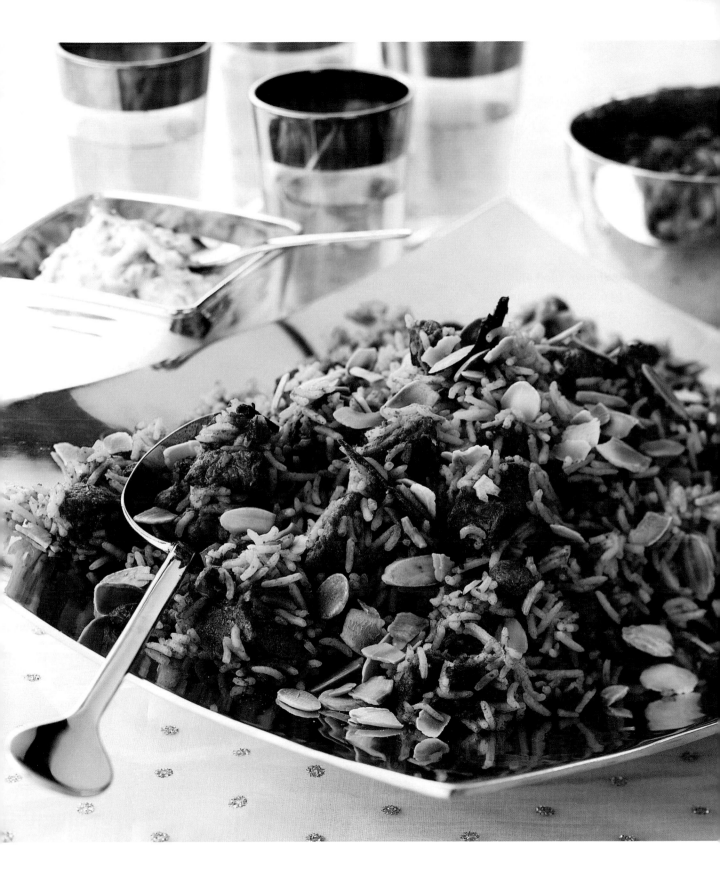

chicken & *cashew pancakes*

Chicken stir-fried with carrots, celery and cabbage, and flavored with orange and sesame, makes a delicious filling for pancakes. The pancakes can be made using a mixture of white and whole-wheat flour, if you like.

SERVES 4 (MAKES 8)   PREPARATION 20 MINUTES   COOKING 30 MINUTES

$3/4$ cup (110 g) all-purpose flour
freshly ground black pepper
1 egg, beaten
$1^1/4$ cups (300 ml) low-fat milk
1 teaspoon (5 ml) canola oil

Chicken and cashew nut filling
$1/3$ cup (50 g) cashew nuts
1 tablespoon (15 ml) canola oil
$2/3$ pound (300 g) boneless, skinless
   chicken breast, cut into strips
1 garlic clove, crushed
1 teaspoon (5 ml) finely chopped
   fresh ginger
1 red chile, seeded and finely
   chopped (optional)
2 carrots, cut into thin sticks
2 celery stalks, cut into thin sticks
grated zest of $1/2$ orange
1 cup (200 g) savoy cabbage,
   shredded
1 tablespoon (15 ml) low-sodium
   soy sauce
1 teaspoon (5 ml) sesame oil

1 To make the pancakes, sift the flour into a bowl and season with a little pepper. Make a well in the center. Combine the egg with the milk, and pour into the well. Gradually whisk the flour into the milk mixture to form a smooth batter.

2 Use a little of the oil to lightly grease an 8 inch (20 cm) nonstick frying pan, and place it over medium heat. Pour in one-eighth of the batter and swirl it evenly across the surface. Cook for 2 minutes, flip the pancake over and cook for about 30 seconds. Slide onto a warm heatproof plate and cover with a sheet of parchment paper.

3 Cook the remaining batter in the same way, making a total of eight pancakes and stacking them up, interleaved with parchment paper. Cover the pancake stack with foil, sealing it well. Place the plate over a saucepan of gently simmering water to keep the pancakes warm.

4 To make the chicken and cashew filling, heat a wok or large frying pan over medium heat. Add the cashews and stir-fry for a few minutes, or until golden. Remove to a plate and set aside.

5 Add the oil to the wok and swirl it around, and add the chicken, garlic, ginger and chile, if using. Stir-fry for 3 minutes, add the carrots and celery and stir-fry for another 2 minutes. Add the orange zest and cabbage and stir-fry for 1 minute. Add the soy sauce and sesame oil and stir-fry for another minute. Return the cashews to the wok and toss to combine.

6 Divide the stir-fry filling among the warm pancakes and fold them over or roll them up. Serve immediately.

Each serving (2 pancakes) provides
405 calories, 28 g protein, 19 g fat
(3 g saturated fat), 31 g carbohydrate
(9 g sugars), 5 g fiber, 332 mg sodium

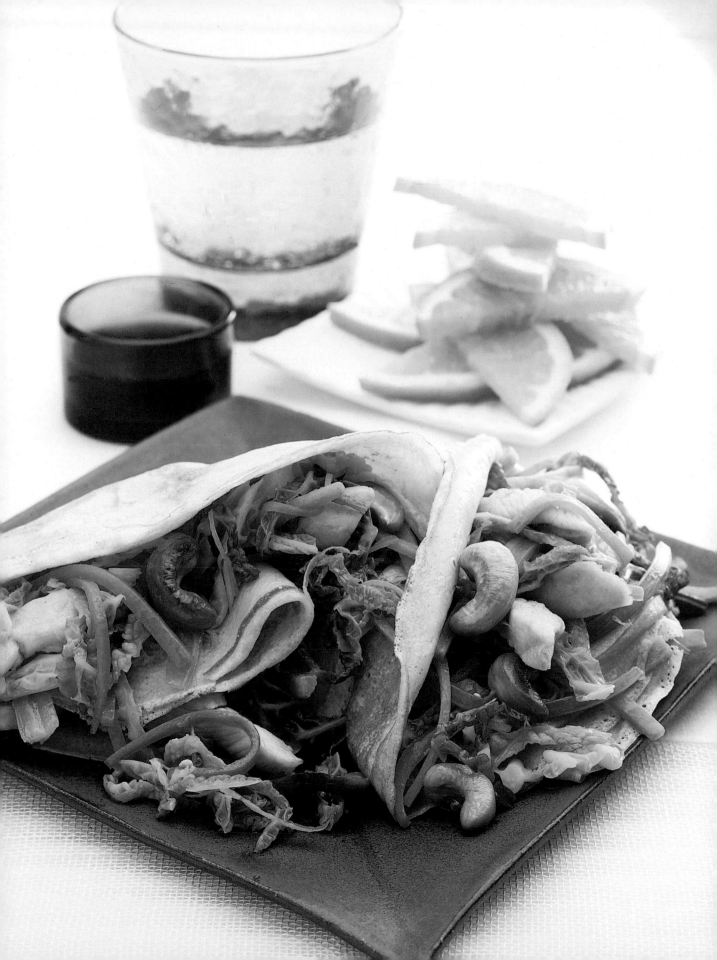

cinnamon-mustard chicken with sweet potatoes & peppers

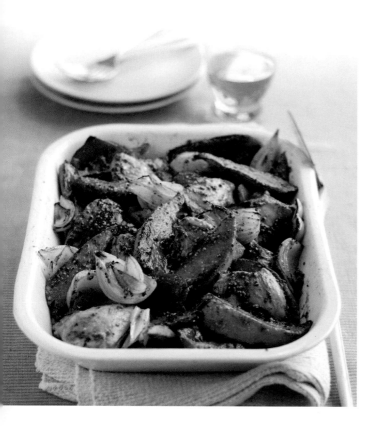

SERVES 4   PREPARATION 10 MINUTES
COOKING 25 MINUTES

2 tablespoons (30 ml) whole-grain mustard
2 teaspoons (10 ml) ground cinnamon
1 cup (200 ml) apple juice
1^1/$_3$ pounds (650 g) boneless, skinless
   chicken thighs
1^2/$_3$ pounds (800 g) sweet potatoes, peeled
   and cut into chunky wedges
4 onions, quartered
2 red peppers, seeds removed and
   quartered lengthwise
2 yellow peppers, seeds removed and
   quartered lengthwise
pinch of salt and freshly ground black pepper
2 tablespoons (30 ml) olive oil

1 Preheat the oven to 465°F (240°C). Put the
   mustard, cinnamon and apple juice in a
   large ovenproof dish or roasting pan and stir
   to combine. Add the chicken, turning the
   pieces over several times to coat in the
   marinade. Set aside.
2 Bring a saucepan of water to a boil, and add
   the sweet potato. Return to a boil and cook
   for 5 minutes, then drain.
3 Add the sweet potatoes to the chicken, along
   with the onions and peppers. Turn all the
   vegetables in the dressing to coat evenly, and
   turn the chicken once more. Season with salt
   and pepper and drizzle with the oil.
4 Roast for 20 minutes, or until the chicken and
   vegetables are cooked and well browned. Test if
   the chicken is cooked by piercing the thickest
   part with the point of a knife; the juices should
   run clear, not pink. Serve immediately.

Each serving provides
519 calories, 37 g protein, 22 g fat
(5 g saturated fat), 44 g carbohydrate
(24 g sugars), 6 g fiber, 336 mg sodium

duck with chestnuts & prunes

SERVES 4   PREPARATION 10 MINUTES
COOKING 15 MINUTES

6 juniper berries
1 tablespoon (30 ml) olive oil
4 boneless, skinless duck breasts, about ¼ pound (125 g) each
1 onion, thinly sliced
2 sprigs fresh rosemary
16 pitted prunes
²/₃ cup (150 g) peeled cooked chestnuts
grated zest of 1 orange
1²/₃ cups (400 ml) red wine
8 orange slices, to garnish

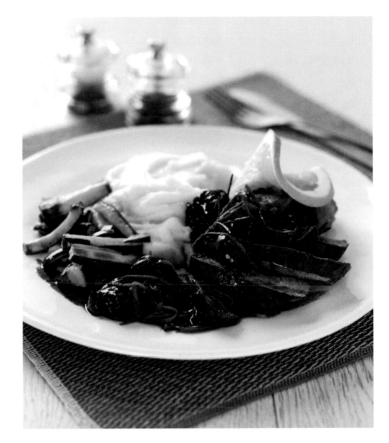

1 Using a rolling pin or mortar and pestle, lightly crush the juniper berries. Set aside.

2 Heat a frying pan over high heat. Add the oil and duck breasts and pan-fry for 1 minute on each side, pressing the duck into the hot pan to brown evenly. Reduce the heat to medium, add the onion and rosemary and cook for 2 minutes. Turn the duck and onions, cover with a lid and cook for another 2 minutes. Transfer to a plate.

3 Add the juniper berries to the pan, along with the prunes, chestnuts and orange zest. Pour in the wine and bring to a boil over high heat. Boil for 3 minutes to reduce the wine a little.

4 Return the duck and onions to the pan with any juices. Reduce the heat to low, cover the pan and simmer for 3 minutes, stirring occasionally. Divide the duck, chestnuts and prunes among four plates. Spoon the sauce on top and garnish with orange slices. Serve with mashed potatoes and steamed zucchini.

COOK'S TIPS

+ *Juniper berries are a dark purple berry, and one of the flavoring ingredients in gin. You will find them in the herb and spice aisle in most large supermarkets.*

+ *Cooked chestnuts are sold in vacuum-packs or cans.*

Each serving provides
406 calories, 27 g protein, 11 g fat (2 g saturated fat), 32 g carbohydrate (14 g sugars), 8 g fiber, 86 mg sodium

hungarian-style *meatballs*

Ground turkey and mushrooms make succulent, low-fat meatballs, simmered in a sauce make with tomato purée and red and green peppers. Paprika adds warmth to the dish and new potatoes turn it into a complete meal.

SERVES 4   PREPARATION 25 MINUTES   COOKING 55 MINUTES

1 tablespoon (15 ml) olive oil
1 small onion, finely chopped
1$^{1}/_{3}$ cups (340 g) mushrooms, finely chopped
$^{2}/_{3}$ pound (340 g) ground turkey
$^{2}/_{3}$ cup (55 g) fresh whole-grain breadcrumbs
1 egg, beaten
2 tablespoons (30 ml) chopped fresh parsley, plus small sprigs, to garnish
freshly ground black pepper
1 pound (550 g) small new potatoes, halved if large
4 tablespoons (60 ml) low-fat plain yogurt

Sauce
2 tablespoons (30 ml) olive oil
1 onion, finely chopped
2 garlic cloves, crushed
1 red pepper, seeded and thinly sliced
1 green pepper, seeded and thinly sliced
1 tablespoon (15 ml) paprika
4 cups (1 liter) tomato purée
pinch of caraway seeds

1 Heat the oil in a large flameproof casserole dish over medium heat. Add the onion and mushrooms and cook, stirring frequently, for about 10 minutes. The mushrooms will give up their liquid initially, but this will evaporate to leave the mixture greatly reduced, dark in color and very thick. Transfer the mushroom mixture to a large bowl and let cool slightly.

2 Add the ground turkey to the bowl and use a fork to break up the pieces. Add the breadcrumbs, egg, parsley and a little pepper. Mix until thoroughly combined. Wet your hands a little to prevent the mixture from sticking to them, and shape the turkey mixture into 20 walnut-sized balls. Set the meatballs aside.

3 Clean the casserole dish and return it to medium heat. To make the sauce, heat the oil in the dish, add the onion and cook for 4–5 minutes, stirring frequently, until softened. Add the garlic and peppers and cook, stirring constantly, for 2–3 minutes. Stir in the paprika and cook for 1 minute, pour in the purée and bring to a boil over high heat.

4 Stir in the caraway seeds and season with pepper. Add the meatballs and potatoes to the simmering sauce. Cover and simmer gently for 35 minutes, or until the potatoes are tender. Ladle the meatballs, potatoes and sauce into bowls. Top each serving with 1 tablespoon (15 ml) of yogurt and a sprig of parsley.

Each serving provides
606 calories, 48 g protein, 23 g fat (5 g saturated fat),
52 g carbohydrate (18 g sugars), 12 g fiber, 311 mg sodium

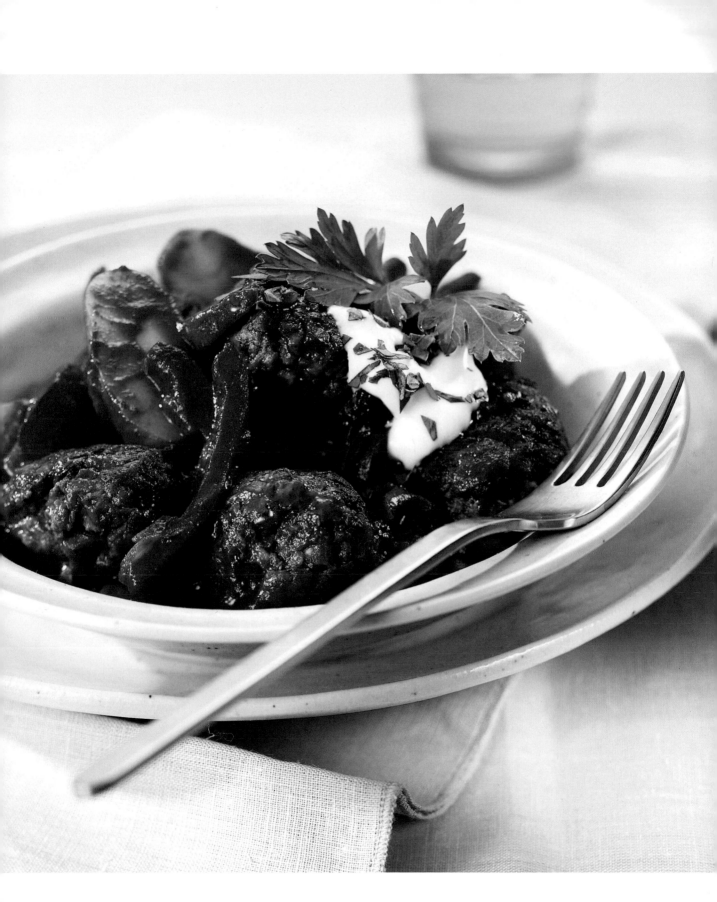

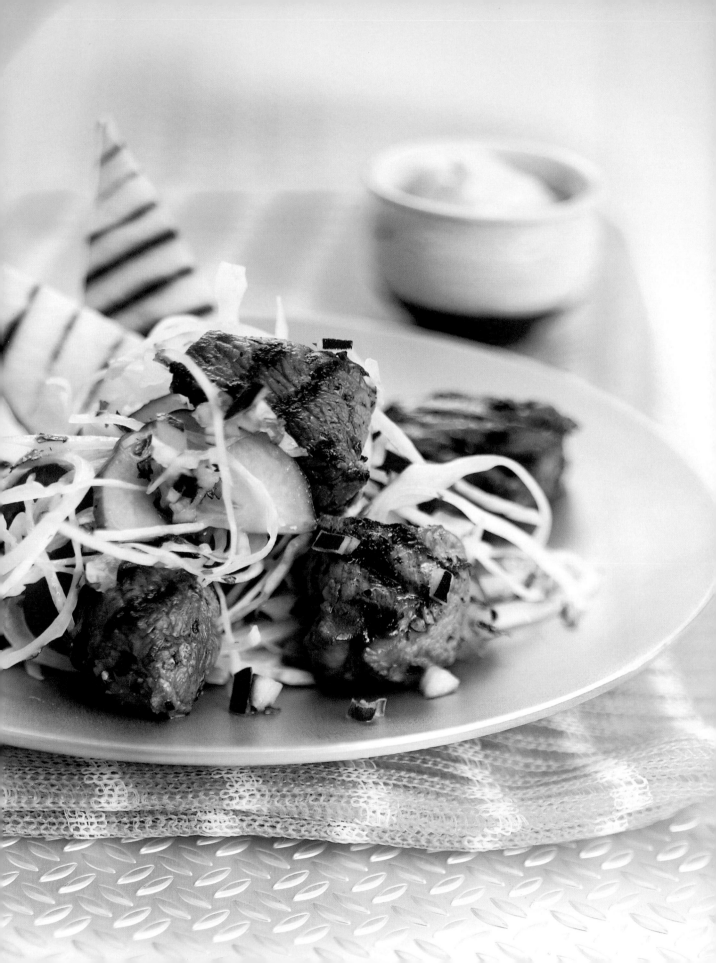

greek *lamb kebabs*

Cubes of lamb flavored with a mixture of garlic, lemon juice and fresh oregano are cooked on skewers and served with pita bread and a Greek-style tomato and cabbage salad for a deliciously aromatic main meal.

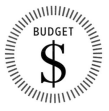

BUDGET
$

SERVES 4   PREPARATION 15 MINUTES   COOKING 10 MINUTES

1$\frac{1}{2}$ tablespoons (22 ml) extra
   virgin olive oil
2 large cloves garlic, crushed
juice of $\frac{1}{2}$ lemon
1 tablespoon (15 ml) chopped
   fresh oregano
1$\frac{1}{4}$ pounds (600 g) boneless leg of
   lamb, trimmed of fat, cut into
   1 inch (2.5 cm) cubes
4 pita breads, cut into triangles
Greek-style yogurt, to serve
   (optional)

Cabbage and tomato salad
6 tomatoes, thickly sliced
1 red onion, finely chopped
1 baby green cabbage, about
   $\frac{1}{2}$ pound (250 g), core removed
   and thinly shredded
$\frac{1}{4}$ cucumber, halved and
   thinly sliced
$\frac{1}{3}$ cup (20 g) chopped fresh mint
juice of $\frac{1}{2}$ lemon
1 tablespoon (15 ml) extra
   virgin olive oil
pinch of salt and freshly
   ground black pepper

1 Place a grill pan over medium heat or preheat the broiler to medium. Put the oil, garlic, lemon juice and oregano in a bowl and stir to mix together. Add the cubes of lamb and turn to coat in the marinade. Thread the lamb onto four skewers.
2 Cook the lamb on the grill pan or under the broiler for 7–8 minutes, or until just cooked through, turning frequently. Briefly warm the pita bread in the pan or under the broiler.
3 Meanwhile, make the cabbage and tomato salad. Put all the ingredients in a bowl, and toss together gently.
4 Serve the kebabs with the salad and pita bread, and with a small dollop of yogurt, if desired.

Each serving provides
475 calories, 37 g protein, 20 g fat (6 g saturated fat), 34 g carbohydrate (9 g sugars), 7 g fiber, 434 mg sodium

LAMB is a rich source of B vitamins, needed for a healthy nervous system. It is also a good source of zinc and iron.

CABBAGE belongs to a family of vegetables that contain a number of different phytochemicals that may help to protect against breast cancer. Cabbage is also a good source of vitamin C and among the richest vegetable sources of folate.

ONIONS, along with leeks, garlic, Jerusalem artichokes, asparagus, barley and bananas, contain a type of dietary fiber called fructooligosaccharides (FOS). This is believed to stimulate the growth of friendly bacteria in the gut while inhibiting the growth of bad bacteria.

quick bulgur salad with lamb

Bulgur is a low-GI grain made from durum wheat and makes an excellent accompaniment to meat or fish dishes. The wheat grains have already been parboiled, so it doesn't take long to prepare.

SERVES 4 PREPARATION 10 MINUTES, PLUS 20 MINUTES SOAKING COOKING 5 MINUTES

1 cup (175 g) bulgur
1¼ cups (300 ml) boiling water
4 scallions, thinly sliced
2 large tomatoes, chopped
1 tablespoon (15 ml) lemon juice
1 tablespoon (15 ml) extra virgin
    olive oil, plus extra for frying
pinch of salt and freshly ground
    black pepper
12 lamb chops, French trimmed

1 Place the bulgur in a heatproof bowl, and pour boiling water over. Cover tightly with foil and set aside for 15–20 minutes, or until the grains are tender and all the water has absorbed. Fluff up the grains with a fork and place in a large salad bowl.

2 Add the scallions, tomatoes and lemon juice to the bulgur. Drizzle with the oil, season with salt and pepper and toss to combine. Set aside.

3 Lightly oil a grill pan or heavy-bottom frying pan and place over medium–high heat. Cook the lamb chops for 2 minutes on each side for medium, and remove from the pan. Serve the lamb chops with the bulgur salad.

COOK'S TIP

+ *Ask your butcher for French-trimmed lamb chops. These have been trimmed of fat, with the bone scraped clean for a nicer look.*

Each serving provides
332 calories, 22 g protein, 14 g fat (4 g saturated fat), 29 g carbohydrate (3 g sugars), 7 g fiber, 217 mg sodium

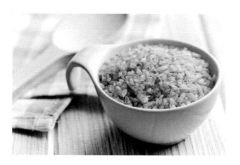

Food Fact

   BULGUR is made by parboiling wheat grains until soft, drying them and then coarsely grinding them. As the grains have already been parboiled, bulgur is very quick to prepare: It can be briefly boiled or, alternatively, left to soak in boiling water until soft. Bulgur is made from the whole wheat grain and is a good source of low-GI carbohydrate, dietary fiber and B vitamins.

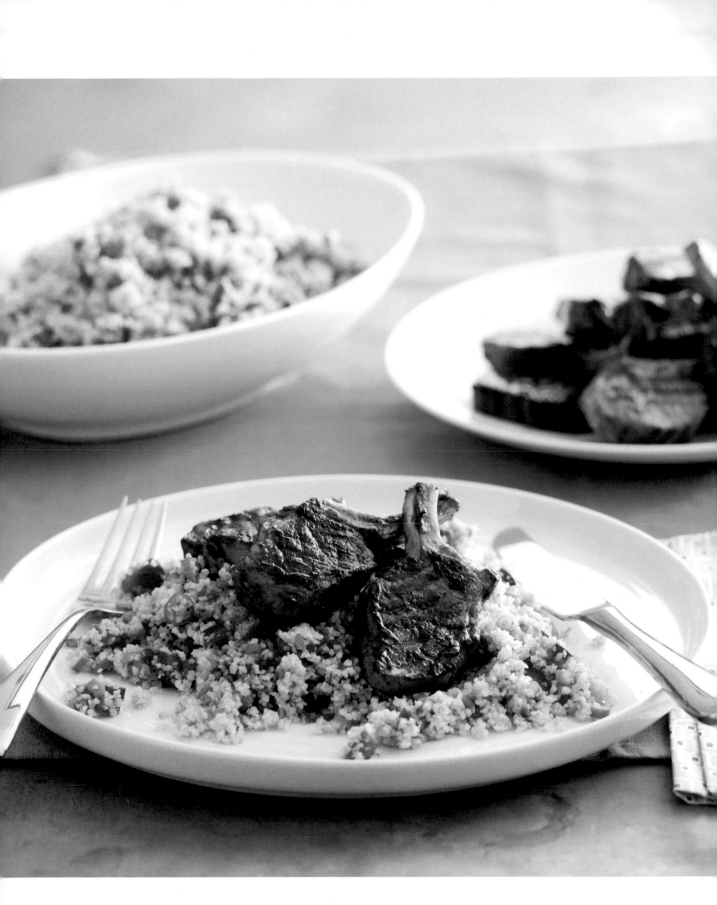

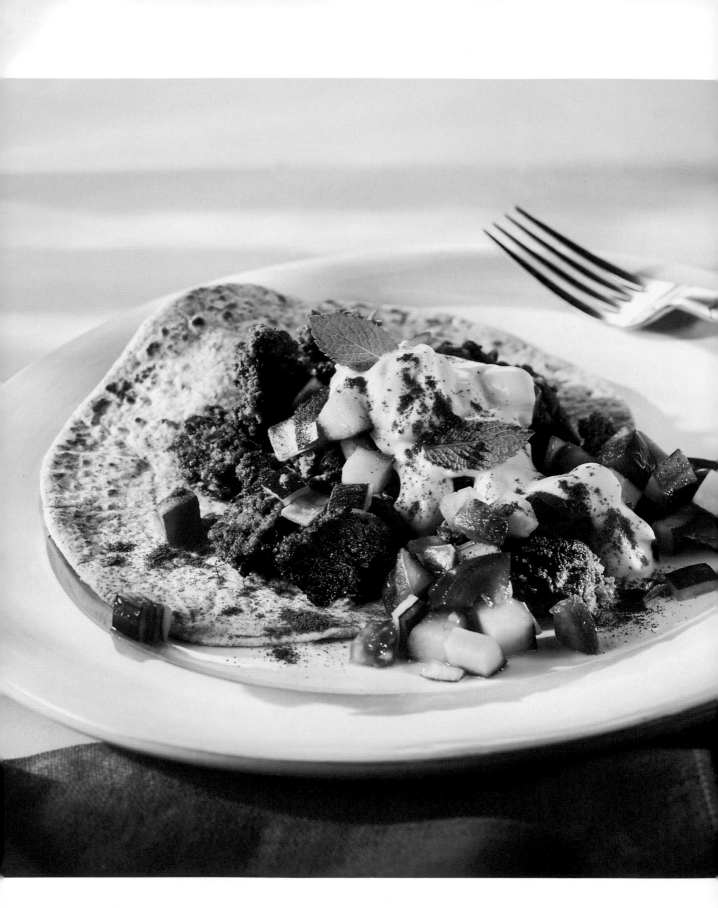

Indian-style baked lamb

This recipe is an Indian version of stuffed pancakes, made with ground lamb marinated in a tempting blend of yogurt, herbs and spices. Green chilies and garam masala—a flavorsome mix of toasted ground spices—add a touch of heat to the dish.

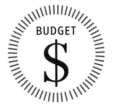

BUDGET
$

SERVES 4   PREPARATION 15 MINUTES, PLUS 1–2 HOURS (OR OVERNIGHT) MARINATING
COOKING 30 MINUTES

1 pound (500 g) lean ground lamb
2 tablespoons (30 ml) olive oil
4 large chapattis
1 small cucumber, diced
1/2 red onion, finely diced
1 tomato, diced
3 tablespoons (45 ml) low-fat
  plain yogurt
paprika, to serve
fresh mint leaves, to serve

Marinade
1/2 cup (125 ml) low-fat plain yogurt
3/4 cup (185 g) chopped onions
2 tablespoons (30 ml) chopped
  fresh ginger
8 cloves garlic, chopped
2 green chilies, seeded and chopped
6 sprigs fresh cilantro, including
  tender stems
6–8 fresh mint leaves or 1/2 teaspoon
  (2 ml) dried mint
pinch of salt
1 teaspoon (5 ml) garam masala
1 tablespoon (15 ml) ground coriander
1 tablespoon (15 ml) ground cumin
1/2 teaspoon (2 ml) ground turmeric

1 To make the marinade, put all the ingredients into a food processor and process to form a smooth purée.

2 Put the ground lamb in a bowl, add the marinade and stir to combine thoroughly. Cover and refrigerate for 1–2 hours, or overnight, if time permits, to allow the flavors to develop. Return the lamb to room temperature before cooking.

3 Preheat the oven to 400°F (200°C). Pour the oil into a large casserole dish, add the lamb and spread it out evenly. Bake in the top half of the oven for 10 minutes.

4 Remove the dish from the oven and break the lamb into chunky pieces with a fork, then stir thoroughly to absorb any cooking juices. Return to the oven and cook for another 15–20 minutes, stirring halfway through, until the lamb is lightly browned and most of the cooking juices have evaporated. Give the lamb a final stir so that any remaining juices are absorbed.

5 Spoon equal portions of lamb on top of each chapatti, and top with some chopped cucumber, onion, tomato and a little yogurt. Serve garnished with a sprinkle of paprika and one or two mint leaves.

Each serving provides
441 calories, 35 g protein, 20 g fat (5 g saturated fat), 32 g carbohydrate (8 g sugars), 8 g fiber, 425 mg sodium

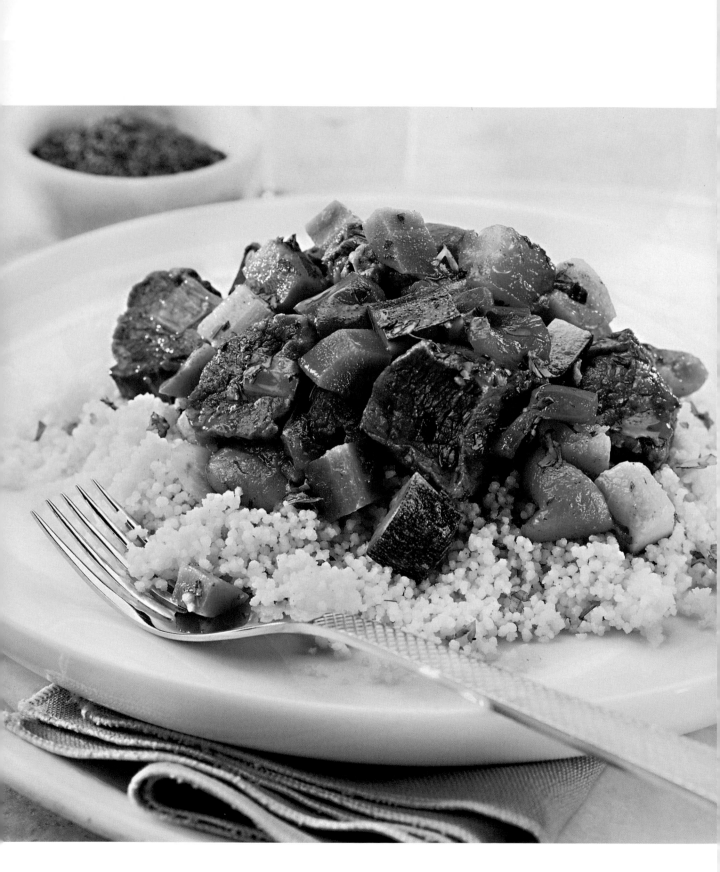

spicy lamb tagine with couscous

Capture the atmosphere of Morocco with this hearty stew of lamb, fruit and vegetables, served with fluffy couscous. The spices used here go particularly well with lamb and help to mellow its sometimes strong flavor, although you could use beef instead if you wish.

SERVES 6   PREPARATION 30 MINUTES   COOKING 2 HOURS

3 tablespoons (45 ml) olive oil

1²/₃ pounds (800 g) lamb leg steak, trimmed and cut into 1 inch (2.5 cm) cubes

1/2 cup (125 g) onions, chopped

2 cloves garlic, chopped

1/2 teaspoon (5 ml) cayenne pepper

1 piece cinnamon stick, 2 inches (5 cm), broken in half

1 teaspoon (5 ml) ground ginger

1 teaspoon (5 ml) paprika

10–12 saffron threads

1/4 teaspoon (1 ml) salt

freshly ground black pepper

2/3 cup (150 g) dried apricots, quartered

3/4 cup (185 g) carrots, diced

1/2 cup (100 g) zucchini, diced

1¹/₂ cups (375 g) tomatoes, chopped

2 tablespoons (30 ml) chopped fresh cilantro leaves, plus extra to serve

2 tablespoons (30 ml) chopped fresh parsley, plus extra to serve

2 cups (375 g) couscous

1 Heat the oil in the bottom of a double boiler or a large saucepan over medium–high heat, add the lamb and cook, stirring, for 2–3 minutes, or until browned. Add the onions, garlic, cayenne pepper, cinnamon, ginger, paprika and saffron to the lamb. Season with half of the salt and some pepper, and add enough water to cover. Bring to a boil, cover the pan, reduce the heat to low and simmer for 1¹/₂ hours.

2 Add the apricots, carrots, zucchini, tomatoes, cilantro and parsley to the pan and cook, covered, for another 15 minutes.

3 Meanwhile, put the couscous into a bowl, add just enough cold water to cover and leave for 5 minutes to absorb the liquid.

4 Transfer the couscous to the top of the double boiler, or if using a saucepan put it in a colander, and steam the couscous over the tagine for 15 minutes, or until fluffy and tender. Season with the remaining salt.

5 To serve, spoon the couscous into a serving dish. Remove the lamb and vegetables from the pan with a slotted spoon and place on top of the couscous. Sprinkle with the extra cilantro and parsley. Pour the broth into a sauce boat and serve separately.

Each serving provides
417 calories, 34 g protein, 18 g fat (5 g saturated fat),
31 g carbohydrate (14 g sugars), 5 g fiber, 215 mg sodium

mini lamb roast
with red wine gravy

A sweet red currant-glazed lamb roast makes a wonderful dinner for two. Here it is served with a red wine gravy and a medley of roasted vegetables.

SERVES 2   PREPARATION 15 MINUTES   COOKING 50 MINUTES

1 boneless lamb mini rump
  roast, ³/₄ pound (400 g)
1¹/₂ tablespoons (22 ml)
  red currant jelly
1 clove garlic, sliced
1 sprig fresh rosemary, leaves only
4 small new potatoes, unpeeled
  and left whole
1 onion, quartered
6 baby carrots, halved lengthwise
  if thick
2 small zucchini, halved lengthwise
2 teaspoons (10 ml) olive oil
freshly ground black pepper

Red wine gravy
3 tablespoons (45 ml) red wine
¹/₂ cup (125 ml) homemade or
  low-sodium chicken stock
2 teaspoons (10 ml) all-purpose flour
2 teaspoons (10 ml) olive oil spread

1 Preheat the oven to 400°F (200°C). Using a small sharp knife, make several deep incisions in the lamb. Brush the red currant jelly over the lamb, and push the garlic slices and rosemary leaves into the slits. Place the lamb in a roasting pan.

2 Put the vegetables in a bowl, drizzle with the oil and turn to coat. Season with pepper, and arrange in the roasting pan, around the lamb. Place in the oven and roast for 35 minutes, or until the lamb is cooked but still slightly pink in the middle.

3 Remove roasting pan from the oven, transfer the lamb to a warm plate and loosely cover with foil. Let rest in a warm place for 5–10 minutes to let the juices settle before carving. If the vegetables are not golden and cooked through, return the pan to the oven and roast the vegetables for another 5–10 minutes, or until tender. Remove to a warm dish and keep warm.

4 To make the red wine gravy, pour the roasting juices and brown bits into a small saucepan. Add the wine and stock and stir over medium heat, then bring to a boil. Combine the flour and olive oil spread, and whisk into the wine and stock mixture. Reduce the heat to low and stir for several minutes, until the sauce thickens into a gravy. Season with pepper. Serve the lamb and roasted vegetables with the gravy.

Each serving provides
607 calories, 52 g protein, 20 g fat (5 g saturated fat),
49 g carbohydrate (22 g sugars), 9 g fiber, 381 mg sodium

pork steaks with
glazed plums & red cabbage

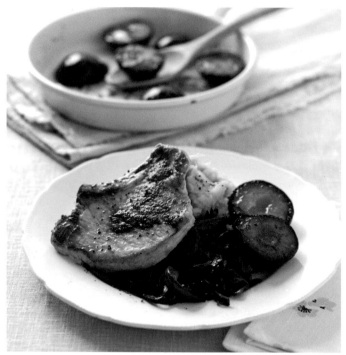

SERVES 4   PREPARATION 10 MINUTES
COOKING 25 MINUTES

2 tablespoons (30 ml) olive oil

4 lean boneless pork loin chops,
   about $1/4$ pound (125 g) each

2 red onions, thinly sliced

$1^2/3$ cups (400 g) red cabbage,
   shredded

pinch of ground cloves or allspice

$1/2$ cup (100 ml) pomegranate
   juice drink

3 tablespoons (45 ml) raw sugar

3 tablespoons (45 ml) red wine
   vinegar

8 ripe plums, halved

freshly ground black pepper

1 Heat the oil in a large frying pan over high heat. Add the pork and cook for 3 minutes on each side, or until browned. Reduce the heat to medium, add the onions and cook for another 5 minutes, stirring occasionally. Transfer the pork to a shallow dish, leaving the onions in the pan.

2 Add the cabbage and ground cloves to the pan and fry, stirring, for 5 minutes. Pour in the pomegranate juice and bring to a boil. Return the pork to the pan with any juices from the dish. Reduce the heat to medium, then cover and cook for 3 minutes. Transfer the pork to four warmed plates.

3 Add 1 tablespoon (15 ml) each of sugar and vinegar to the cabbage and boil for 30 seconds, stirring, to glaze the cabbage. Divide the cabbage among the plates of pork.

4 Add the plums to the pan, placing them cut sides down. Sprinkle the remaining 2 tablespoons (30 ml) each of sugar and vinegar over the plums and cook over high heat for 4 minutes, shaking the pan so the sugar dissolves. Season to taste with pepper and divide the plums and their glaze among the plates and serve.

Each serving provides
416 calories, 30 g protein, 18 g fat
(6 g saturated fat), 32 g carbohydrate
(29 g sugars), 7 g fiber, 82 mg sodium

pork with *fruit relish*

SERVES 4 PREPARATION 20 MINUTES,
PLUS COOLING COOKING 15 MINUTES

1 tablespoon (15 ml) balsamic
   vinegar
1 tablespoon (15 ml) Dijon mustard
4 lean pork loin cutlets or chops,
   about $1/2$ pound (200 g) each,
   patted dry with paper towels
freshly ground black pepper
2 tablespoons (30 ml) olive oil
$3/4$ pound (400 g) broccolini or
   asparagus spears
$1^2/_3$ cups (400 g) quinoa, rinsed
   and cooked (see page 61)

Apple and blueberry relish
2 green apples, such as granny
   smith, peeled, cored and diced
1 small onion, finely diced
$1/3$ cup (80 ml) balsamic vinegar
$1/4$ cup (50 g) soft brown sugar
2 cloves
$1/2$ cup (125 g) fresh blueberries

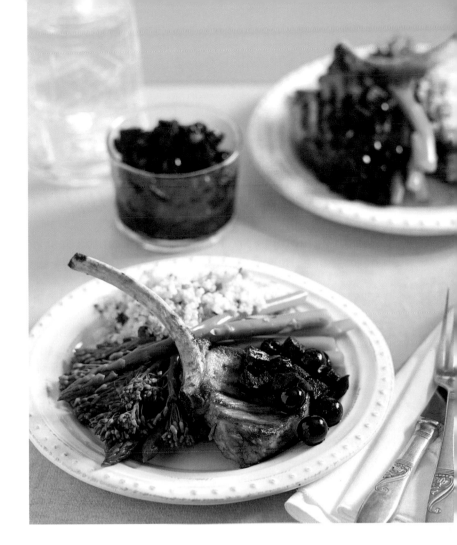

1 Combine the vinegar and mustard
   in a small bowl. Brush both sides
   of the pork with the mustard
   mixture and season with pepper.
   Set aside to marinate.
2 To make the apple and blueberry
   relish, put the apples, onion,
   vinegar, sugar and cloves in a
   saucepan over medium heat and
   stir to combine. Bring to a boil,
   stirring to dissolve the sugar.
   Reduce the heat to low and simmer
   for about 4 minutes, or until the

apples and onion are just tender. Add the blueberries,
simmer for another 3–4 minutes, until blueberries have
softened. Remove from heat, discard cloves; let cool.

3 Heat a grill pan or frying pan over high heat. Add the
   oil, then add the pork. Reduce the heat to medium and
   cook for 3–4 minutes, depending on thickness, until
   small beads of moisture appear on the top of each pork
   chop; do not turn before then. Turn and cook the other
   side until done to your liking (1–2 minutes for rare,
   2–3 minutes for medium and 3–4 minutes for well
   done). Remove from heat and let rest for 3–4 minutes.
4 Steam the broccolini over a saucepan of boiling water
   for about 5 minutes, or until just tender. Serve the pork
   with the quinoa, broccolini and a spoonful of apple and
   blueberry relish on the side.

Each serving provides
607 calories, 50 g protein, 20 g fat (5 g saturated fat),
57 g carbohydrate (30 g sugars), 6 g fiber, 287 mg sodium

pan-fried *pork chops*

This classic pairing of pork served with braised red cabbage and apple is big on flavor as well as packed with vitamins and fiber. Replacing the boiled potato with a sweet potato lowers the GI of this meal.

SERVES
2

SERVES 2   PREPARATION 15 MINUTES   COOKING 15 MINUTES

4 small new potatoes, about
  $1/2$ pound (250 g), halved
2 teaspoons (10 ml) vegetable oil
2 pork cutlets, about 5 ounces
  (160 g) each
3 teaspoons (15 ml) olive oil spread
1 green apple, peeled, cored and
  thinly sliced
$1^1/2$ cups (115 g) finely shredded
  red cabbage
pinch of caraway seeds
$1/2$ teaspoon (2 ml) soft brown sugar
$1/2$ teaspoon (2 ml) red wine vinegar
pinch of salt and freshly ground
  black pepper
2 tablespoons (30 ml) chopped
  fresh parsley

1 Place the potatoes in a saucepan and cover with water. Cover and bring to a boil over medium–high heat, tilt the lid so the pan is partially covered and cook for 10 minutes, or until the potatoes are tender.
2 Meanwhile, heat the oil in a nonstick frying pan over medium heat. Add the pork and cook for 4 minutes on each side, or until browned and cooked through. Transfer to a warm plate and cover loosely with foil.
3 Melt half of the olive oil spread in the same frying pan. Add the apple and cook for 2 minutes, turning once, then add the cabbage and caraway seeds. Cook, stirring, for 5 minutes, or until the cabbage is soft. Stir in the sugar and vinegar, and season with salt and pepper.
4 Drain the potatoes and toss with the remaining olive oil spread and the parsley. Season with salt and pepper. Serve the pork with the potatoes and cabbage.

Each serving provides
401 calories, 37 g protein, 16 g fat (4 g saturated fat),
27 g carbohydrate (11 g sugars), 6 g fiber, 448 mg sodium

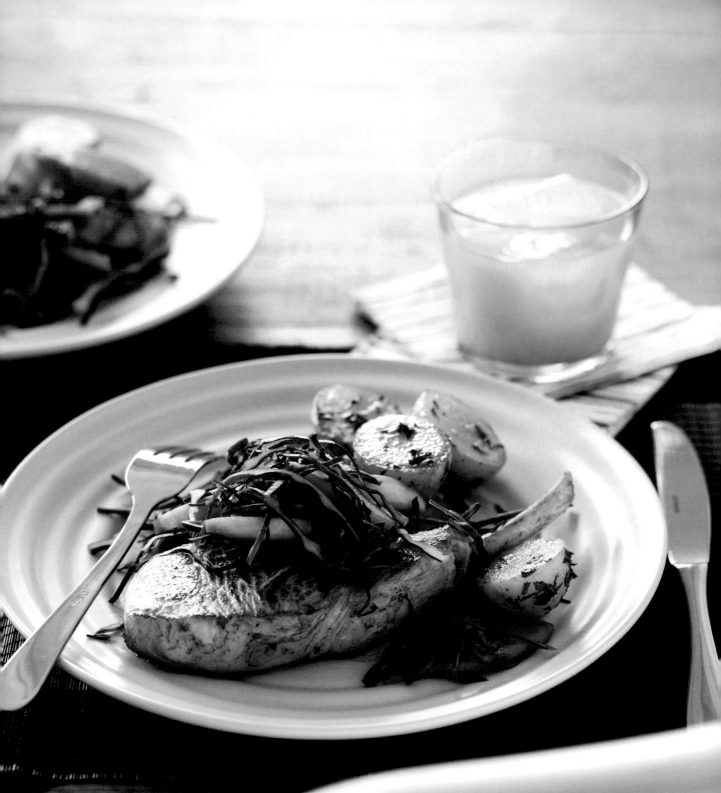

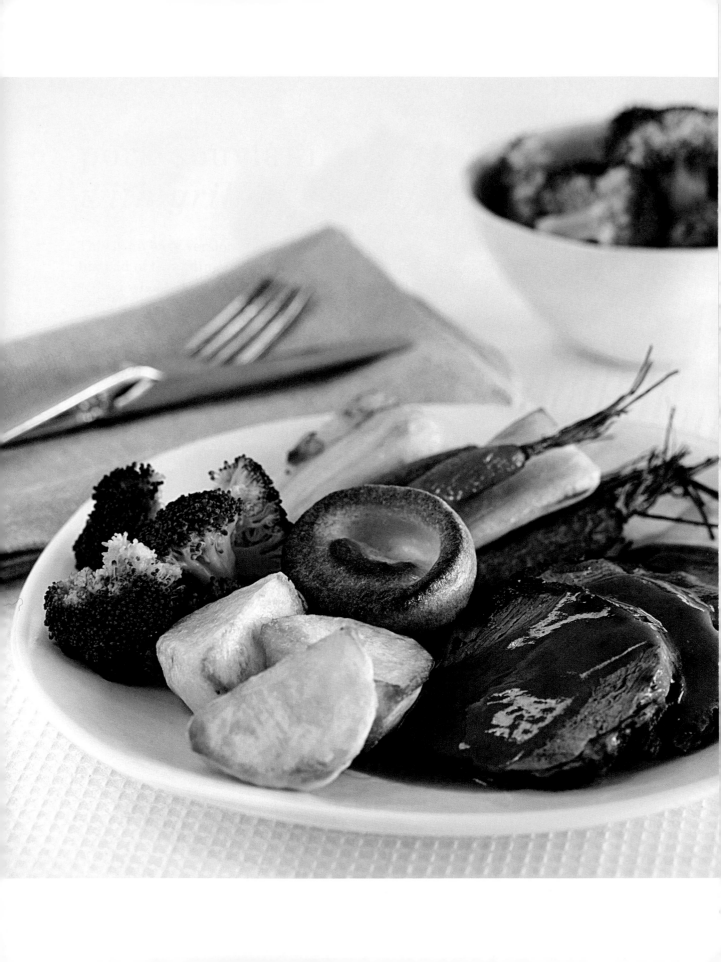

sunday special *roast beef*

Succulent roast beef, crispy roast potatoes, root vegetables and feather-light, old-fashioned Yorkshire puddings make one of the best-loved Sunday dinners.

SERVES 8 PREPARATION 20 MINUTES COOKING 2¼ HOURS

3 pounds (1.5 kg) boned, rolled and tied lean sirloin of beef, trimmed of fat
freshly ground black pepper
4 teaspoons (20 ml) English mustard
3 pounds (1.5 kg) potatoes, such as russet or Yukon gold, peeled and cut into chunks
1⅓ pounds (650 g) baby parsnips, halved lengthwise
1⅓ pounds (650 g) carrots, halved lengthwise
3 tablespoons (45 ml) sunflower oil
1¾ cups (450 ml) homemade or low-sodium beef stock
steamed broccoli florets, to serve

Yorkshire puddings
½ cup (75 g) all-purpose flour
1 egg, lightly beaten
⅓ cup (100 ml) low-fat milk
1 tablespoon (15 ml) sunflower oil

1 Preheat the oven to 350°F (180°C). Put the beef, fat side up, on a rack in a large roasting pan. Season with pepper, and spread with 3 teaspoons (15 ml) of the mustard. For rare, roast the beef for 1 hour 20 minutes; for medium, 1 hour 40 minutes; for well done, 2 hours. Baste occasionally with the juices in the pan.

2 Meanwhile, prepare the Yorkshire pudding batter. Put the flour in a bowl, make a well in the center and add the egg. Add a little of the milk and beat together, gradually working in the flour. Slowly beat in the remaining milk and ⅓ cup (75 ml) water until all the flour is incorporated and the batter is smooth. Set aside.

3 Cook the potatoes in a large saucepan of boiling water for 5 minutes, and drain. Boil the parsnips and carrots for 3 minutes, and drain.

4 One hour before the end of roasting time for the beef, coat the vegetables in 3 tablespoons (45 ml) of oil and place in a nonstick roasting pan in the oven. Turn the vegetables after 30 minutes. When cooked, remove the roast from the oven, place on a plate and cover loosely with foil. Remove vegetables and cover to keep warm.

5 Increase the heat to 425°F (220°C). Grease eight cups of a nonstick muffin pan with oil. Place the pan in the top of the oven to heat for 3 minutes, then pour in the batter and bake for 15 minutes, or until golden.

6 Meanwhile, to make the gravy, slowly pour the fat out of the roasting pan, leaving the caramelized bits behind. Place the pan on the stovetop over medium heat, add the stock and bring to a boil, stirring to loosen the brown bits; simmer until slightly reduced. Season with pepper and stir in the remaining mustard and any beef juices that have collected on the plate; skim off any fat. Place the meat on a platter and surround with the vegetables and Yorkshire puddings. Pour the gravy into a gravy boat and serve.

Each serving provides
579 calories, 49 g protein, 22 g fat (6 g saturated fat), 45 g carbohydrate (10 g sugars), 8 g fiber, 414 mg sodium

beef & pepper burgers

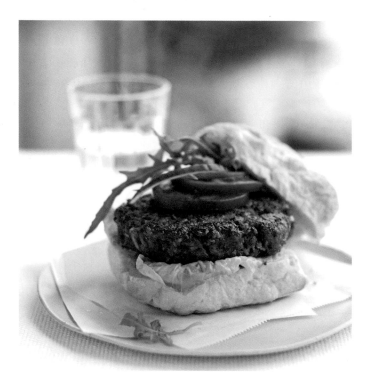

SERVES 4   PREPARATION 15 MINUTES
COOKING 15 MINUTES

1 egg
1 slice whole-grain bread
2 large carrots, finely grated
2 scallions, thinly sliced
1 small red pepper, finely chopped
2 cloves garlic, crushed
1 teaspoon (5 ml) dried oregano
2 tablespoons (30 ml) tomato purée
1/2 cup (50 g) rolled oats
1/2 pound (250 g) lean ground beef
1 tablespoon (15 ml) sunflower oil
4 burger buns
lettuce, tomato, arugula and onion,
   to serve

1 Preheat the broiler to medium–high. Line a broiler pan with foil. Beat the egg in a large bowl. Add the bread and turn it in the egg a couple of times. Add the carrots, scallions, pepper and garlic to the bowl, but don't mix in.

2 Add the oregano and tomato purée, and stir to combine, breaking up the bread. Mix in the oats and ground beef, and use your hands to squeeze, knead and thoroughly bind all the ingredients together.

3 Divide the beef mixture into four and shape each portion into 4 inch (10 cm) burgers by first rolling into balls, then patting them flat. Place the burgers on the pan and brush with 2 teaspoons (10 ml) of oil. Grill for 7 minutes, or until sizzling and browned. Carefully turn using a large spatula, brush with the remaining oil and cook for another 7 minutes.

4 Split the buns and top with lettuce, a burger, some sliced tomato, arugula and a slice of onion.

OTHER IDEAS

+ *Use pork or lamb instead of ground beef, although lamb has a higher fat content.*
+ *Try skinned venison sausages instead of ground beef for a richly flavored low-fat alternative.*

Each serving provides
359 calories, 22 g protein, 13 g fat
(3 g saturated fat), 36 g carbohydrate
(5 g sugars), 6 g fiber, 411 mg sodium

beef & *bean chili*

SERVES 4   PREPARATION 10 MINUTES
COOKING 25 MINUTES

2$\frac{1}{2}$ tablespoons (37 ml) vegetable oil

1 onion, chopped

1 small red pepper, seeded and
 chopped

1 pound (500 g) lean ground beef

1 tablespoon (15 ml) paprika

1 tablespoon (15 ml) ground cumin

3 cloves garlic, crushed

1 small red chile, seeded
 and chopped

14$\frac{1}{2}$ ounce (400 ml) can no-salt
 diced tomatoes

2 teaspoons (10 ml) tomato paste

1 teaspoon (5 ml) dried oregano

$\frac{1}{2}$ cup (125 ml) red wine or
 low-sodium beef stock

$\frac{1}{2}$ teaspoon (2 ml) sugar

15 ounce (425 ml) can no-salt red
 kidney beans, drained and rinsed

8 small flour tortillas

sour cream, to serve

2 scallions, chopped (optional)

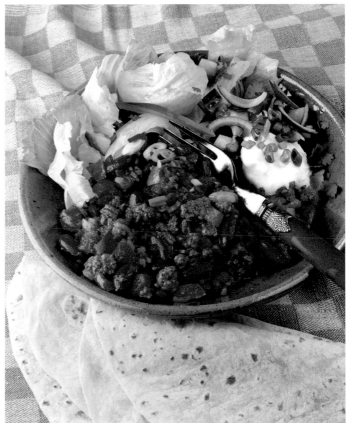

1 Heat the oil in a large flameproof
 casserole dish and fry the onion,
 pepper, ground beef, paprika
 and cumin over medium heat for
 5 minutes, or until browned, stirring
 occasionally to break up any lumps.

2 Add the garlic, chile, tomatoes,
 tomato paste, oregano, wine and
 sugar. Bring to a boil, reduce the
 heat, cover with a lid and simmer
 for 15 minutes.

3 Preheat the broiler to high. Stir the kidney beans into
 the beef mixture and cook for another 5 minutes.
 Meanwhile, place the tortillas under the hot broiler
 for 1 minute, or until warmed through.

4 Transfer the chili to four serving bowls. Top with
 a dollop of sour cream and sprinkle with the
 scallions, if using. Serve with the warmed tortillas,
 and a green salad, if you like.

Each serving provides
475 calories, 33 g protein, 23 g fat (6 g saturated fat),
28 g carbohydrate (7 g sugars), 8 g fiber, 243 mg sodium

hoisin beef *stir-fry*

SERVES 2 PREPARATION 15 MINUTES COOKING 10 MINUTES

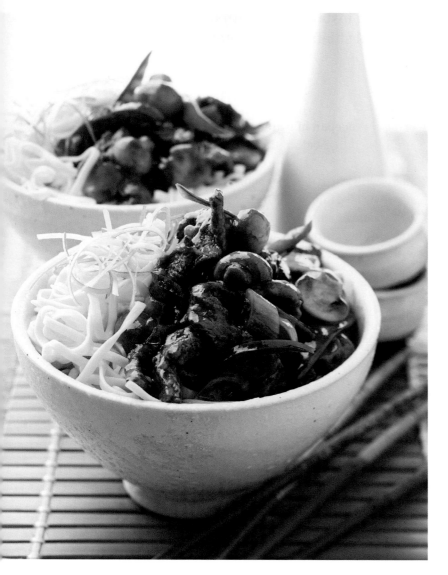

$^{3}/_{4}$ cup (170 g) dried egg noodles
1 tablespoon (15 ml) sunflower oil
2 large cloves garlic, finely shredded
1 teaspoon (5 ml) grated fresh ginger
1 large red pepper, seeded and
    thinly sliced
$^{1}/_{2}$ cup (125 g) small button
    mushrooms, halved
1 sirloin steak, about $^{1}/_{2}$ pound
    (200 g), trimmed of fat and cut
    into thin strips
$^{1}/_{2}$ cup (85 g) snow peas, halved
    lengthwise
4 scallions, sliced
1 tablespoon (15 ml) hoisin sauce
2 teaspoons (10 ml) light soy sauce
$^{1}/_{2}$ teaspoon (2 ml) sesame oil
    (optional)
shredded scallions, to garnish

1 Prepare the noodles according to
   the package instructions.
2 Meanwhile, heat the oil in a wok
   or large frying pan over medium
   heat, add the garlic and ginger and
   cook briefly to release their flavor.
   Add the pepper and mushrooms
   and stir-fry over high heat
   for 2–3 minutes, or until the
   vegetables are starting to soften.
3 Add the strips of steak, snow peas
   and the scallions and stir-fry for
   another 1–2 minutes, or until the
   meat just turns from pink to brown.
4 Add the hoisin sauce, soy sauce
   and 2 tablespoons (30 ml) water
   to the wok and stir well until
   bubbling; drizzle with sesame oil,
   if using. Drain the noodles. Serve
   the stir-fry on the noodles and
   garnish with the scallions.

Each serving provides
521 calories, 34 g protein, 18 g fat (4 g saturated fat),
56 g carbohydrate (10 g sugars), 7 g fiber, 421 mg sodium

roasted eggplant, sweet potatoes & *quinoa with beef*

SERVES 4   PREPARATION 15 MINUTES, PLUS
STANDING   COOKING 20 MINUTES

$1/2$ cup (100 g) red quinoa, rinsed

$1/2$ cup (100 g) white quinoa, rinsed

2 small eggplants, chopped

1 small orange sweet potato, chopped

2 tablespoons (30 ml) olive oil

2 teaspoons (10 ml) ground cardamom

2 teaspoons (10 ml) ground cumin

$2/3$ pound (300 g) thick-cut sirloin or rump steak

$1/2$ cup (60 g) dried cranberries, roughly chopped

$1/4$ cup (50 g) pine nuts, toasted

$1/2$ cup (15 g) fresh cilantro leaves

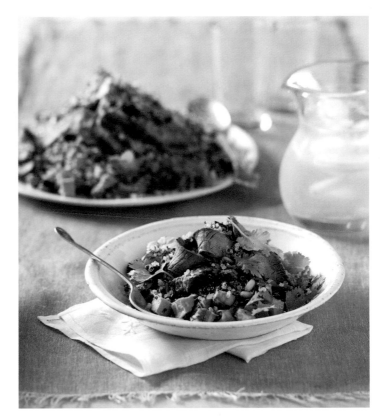

1 Preheat the oven to 400°F (200°C). Line a baking pan with parchment paper.

2 Put both quinoas in a heavy-bottom saucepan with 2 cups (500 ml) water. Bring to a boil, cover, reduce the heat to low and cook for 12–15 minutes, or until the water has evaporated. Turn off the heat and let stand, covered, for 10 minutes.

3 Spread the eggplant and sweet potatoes on the tray. Drizzle with $1^{1}/2$ tablespoons (22 ml) of oil and sprinkle with the cardamom and cumin. Roast for 10–15 minutes, or until golden and cooked through.

4 Heat a grill pan over high heat. Brush the steak with the remaining oil and cook until small beads of moisture appear on top. Turn and cook for another 2–3 minutes, or until cooked to your liking. Remove steak from heat, cover loosely with foil and keep warm. Let rest for 5 minutes.

5 Put the quinoa in a bowl and fluff with a fork. Add the eggplant, sweet potatoes, cranberries, pine nuts and cilantro and toss to combine. Slice the steak very thinly. Divide the quinoa and vegetable mixture among four serving plates, top with the steak and serve.

Each serving provides
539 calories, 27 g protein, 24 g fat (7 g saturated fat), 56 g carbohydrate (10 g sugars), 13 g fiber, 56 mg sodium

veal goulash

SERVES 4   PREPARATION 20 MINUTES
COOKING 1¾ HOURS

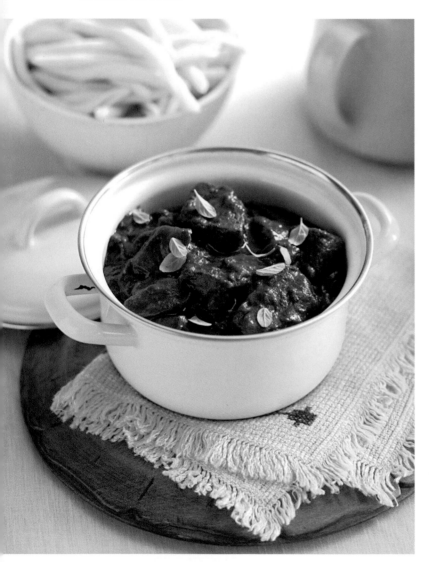

2 pounds (1 kg) boneless veal shoulder
3½ tablespoons (52 ml) olive oil
2 large onions, halved and thinly sliced
2 cloves garlic, chopped
2 large red peppers, cut into chunks
2 tablespoons (30 ml) sweet paprika
2 teaspoons (10 ml) hot paprika
   (optional)
1 tablespoon (15 ml) caraway seeds
2 tablespoons (30 ml) all-purpose flour
2¾ cups (650 ml) no-salt tomato purée
1 cup (250 ml) homemade or low-
   sodium beef stock
1 teaspoon (5 ml) dried marjoram or
   oregano, plus a few fresh leaves, to
   garnish (optional)

1 Trim the veal of any fat or sinew, and
cut it into 1½ inch (3 cm) cubes. Heat
a large frying pan over medium heat,
add 2 tablespoons (30 ml) of the oil,
add the veal in batches and cook until
browned. Set aside.

2 Heat the remaining oil in a large deep
saucepan over medium–low heat.
Add the onions, garlic and peppers
and cook, stirring occasionally, for
2 minutes, or until the onions are soft.
Add the paprika and caraway seeds.
Stir for 30 seconds, add the flour and
stir for 1 minute.

3 Stir in the tomato purée, stock and
marjoram and bring to a boil, then
reduce the heat to low. Add the veal
and simmer, uncovered, for 1½ hours,
or until the veal is tender, stirring
occasionally and adding a little more
stock or water if needed to keep the
veal covered. Serve with noodles or
boiled new potatoes.

Each serving provides
560 calories, 66 g protein, 21 g fat
(4 g saturated fat), 28 g carbohydrate
(15 g sugars), 8 g fiber, 396 mg sodium

veal schnitzels with *coleslaw*

SERVES 4   PREPARATION 20 MINUTES,
PLUS 10 MINUTES CHILLING
COOKING 20 MINUTES

4 veal scallops, about
   $^{1}/_{4}$ pound (100 g) each
1 cup (150 g) all-purpose flour
1 egg, lightly beaten
$^{1}/_{3}$ cup (80 ml) low-fat milk
1 cup (85 g) dry whole-grain
   breadcrumbs
3 teaspoons (15 ml) herb and
   garlic seasoning
olive oil cooking spray
1 lemon, quartered, to serve

Coleslaw
$1^{1}/_{3}$ cups (350 g) red cabbage,
   finely shredded
1 carrot, grated
2 celery stalks, sliced diagonally
1 apple, cored and thinly sliced
$^{1}/_{2}$ cup (125 ml) low-fat plain yogurt
3 tablespoons (45 ml) low-fat mayonnaise
juice of 1 lemon

1 Put each piece of veal between two
   sheets of plastic wrap and pound with
   a meat mallet or rolling pin until about
   $^{1}/_{4}$ inch (0.5 cm) thick.
2 Preheat the oven to 400°F (200°C).
   Put flour on a large plate. Mix egg and
   milk in a bowl. Combine breadcrumbs
   and herb and garlic seasoning on a
   large plate.
3 Coat each veal scallop in flour, shaking
   off any excess. Dip veal in the milk
   mixture, press into breadcrumbs,
   shaking off any excess. Put breaded

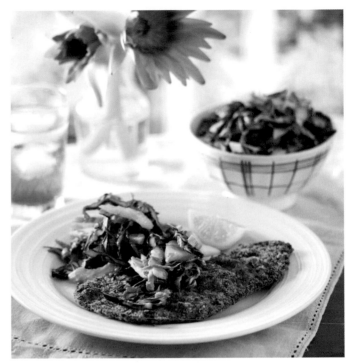

veal on a tray and refrigerate for 10 minutes.
4 Line a large baking pan with foil. Put a wire rack
   on the pan and spray the rack with cooking spray.
   Put veal on the rack and generously spray with
   cooking spray. Bake for 8–10 minutes. Turn the veal
   and spray the other side; cook for another 8–10
   minutes, or until breading is golden and crisp.
5 Meanwhile, to make the coleslaw, combine the
   cabbage, carrot, celery and apple in a large bowl.
   Combine the yogurt, mayonnaise and lemon juice
   in a small bowl, add to the cabbage and toss
   thoroughly. Serve the veal schnitzels with the
   coleslaw and lemon wedges.

Each serving provides
456 calories, 38 g protein, 8 g fat (2 g saturated fat),
57 g carbohydrate (14 g sugars), 8 g fiber, 375 mg sodium

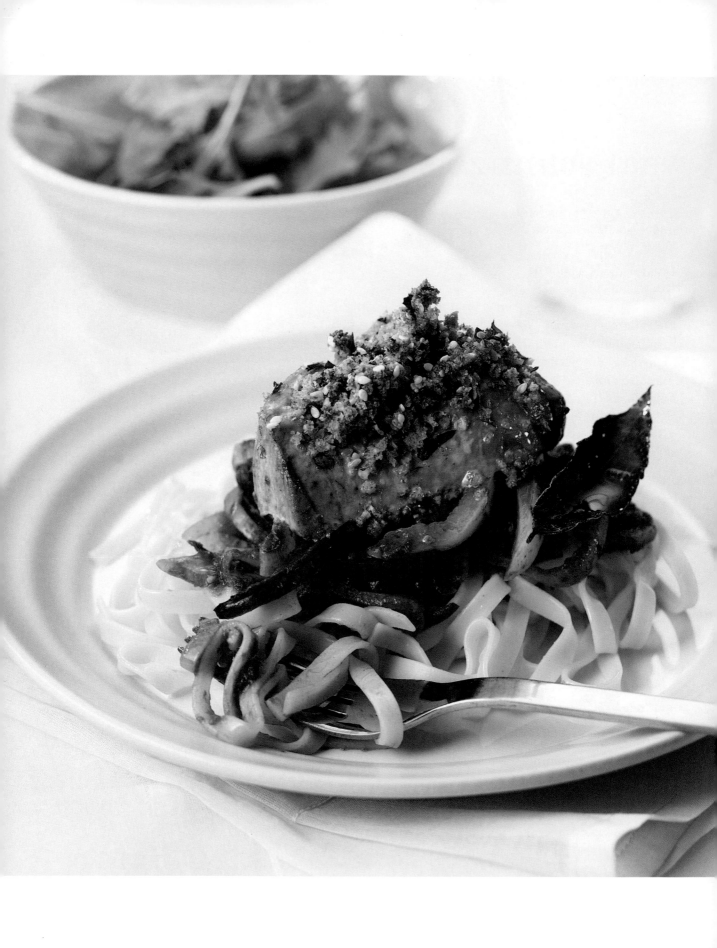

anchovy & sesame-topped tuna

Peppers, tomatoes and a touch of chile make a zesty combination and a perfect partner to these tuna steaks, which are baked with a crisp topping. Tagliatelle is a good accompaniment, along with a crisp green salad or lightly steamed broccoli.

SERVES 4   PREPARATION 15 MINUTES   COOKING 20 MINUTES

1½ tablespoons (22 ml) extra virgin olive oil

1 large onion, thinly sliced

1 large red pepper, seeded and thinly sliced

1 large yellow pepper, seeded and thinly sliced

2 cloves garlic, finely chopped

14½ ounce (400 ml) can no-salt diced tomatoes

1 tablespoon (15 ml) tomato paste

1 bay leaf

½ teaspoon (2 ml) chili paste

2 large tuna steaks, 1 inch (2.5 cm) thick, about 1 pound (500 g) total

freshly ground black pepper

½ pound (250 g) tagliatelle

Anchovy and sesame topping

⅔ cup (55 g) fresh whole-grain breadcrumbs

1 clove garlic

4 anchovy fillets, drained

⅓ cup (10 g) fresh parsley

2 tablespoons (30 ml) sesame seeds

2 teaspoons (10 ml) extra virgin olive oil

1 Preheat the oven to 400°F (200°C). Heat the oil in a frying pan or wide saucepan over a medium heat, and add the onion, peppers and garlic. Cover and cook, stirring frequently, for 3–4 minutes, or until the onion has softened. Stir in the tomatoes, tomato paste, bay leaf and chili paste. Cover the pan again and cook, stirring frequently, for about 7 minutes, or until the peppers are just tender.

2 Meanwhile, to make the anchovy and sesame topping, combine all the ingredients in a food processor and process until finely chopped. Alternatively, chop the breadcrumbs, garlic, anchovies and parsley together, put them in a bowl and mix in the sesame seeds and oil with a fork until well combined.

3 Transfer the pepper mixture to an ovenproof dish large enough to hold the fish in one layer. Season the tuna steaks with pepper and cut each one in half. Lay the four pieces of tuna in the dish and spoon over the topping to cover them evenly. Bake for 10 minutes, or until the fish is just cooked; it will still be a little pink in the center. If you prefer the tuna well done, cook for another 1–2 minutes.

4 Meanwhile, cook the pasta in a saucepan of boiling water for about 10 minutes, or until al dente. Drain and divide among four plates. To serve, top the pasta with some of the pepper mixture and a piece of tuna.

Each serving provides
626 calories, 46 g protein, 22 g fat (5 g saturated fat), 61 g carbohydrate (9 g sugars), 7 g fiber, 426 mg sodium

steamed fish fillets
with spring vegetables

Bamboo steamer baskets are very handy for this recipe—you can stack them so that everything can be steamed together—and the moist heat from steaming prevents the fish from drying out. If using a purchased fish stock, dilute it a little, as the stock will get some extra saltiness and flavor from the soy marinade.

SERVES 4   PREPARATION 15 MINUTES   COOKING 15 MINUTES

4 sea bass fillets, 1^1/$_2$ inches (3.5 cm) thick with skin on, about 5 ounces (150 g) each
3 cups (750 ml) homemade or low-sodium fish stock
1 cup (185 g) couscous
1 strip of lemon zest
1^1/$_2$ cups (350 g) baby carrots
12 scallions, trimmed to about 4 inches (10 cm) long
^{1}/$_2$ pound (200 g) asparagus, trimmed and halved diagonally
2 tablespoons (30 ml) fresh parsley
freshly ground black pepper

Marinade
1 teaspoon (5 ml) grated fresh ginger
1 tablespoon (15 ml) low-sodium soy sauce
^{1}/$_2$ teaspoon (2 ml) sesame oil
1 clove garlic, finely chopped
1 tablespoon (15 ml) dry sherry, dry white wine or vermouth

Each serving provides
382 calories, 39 g protein, 4 g fat (1 g saturated fat), 44 g carbohydrate (8 g sugars), 5 g fiber, 431 mg sodium

1 To make the marinade, combine the ginger, soy sauce, sesame oil, garlic and sherry in a large bowl. Add the fish and turn to coat in the marinade. Set aside.

2 Bring 1 cup (250 ml) of the stock to a boil in a saucepan that will accommodate a steamer basket. Put the couscous in a bowl and pour in the hot stock. Cover and let stand for about 15 minutes, or until the couscous has swelled and absorbed the liquid.

3 Pour the remaining stock into the saucepan. Add the lemon zest and bring to a boil. Add the carrots to the pan, and reduce the heat so the stock is simmering.

4 Place the fish, skin side down, in a single layer in a steamer basket. Add the scallions and asparagus (or put them in a second steamer basket, which will stack on top of the first). Place the steamer basket over the stock and cover. Steam for 10–12 minutes, or until the fish is opaque throughout and begins to flake, and the vegetables are tender.

5 When the couscous is ready, add the chopped parsley and fluff the grains with a fork to combine the couscous and parsley. Season to taste with pepper.

6 Remove the steamer basket from the pan. Drain the carrots, reserving the cooking stock. Divide the couscous among warm plates, and arrange the fish, carrots and steamed vegetables on top. Discard the lemon zest from the cooking stock. Moisten the fish, vegetables and couscous with a little of the stock, and serve with any remaining stock as a sauce.

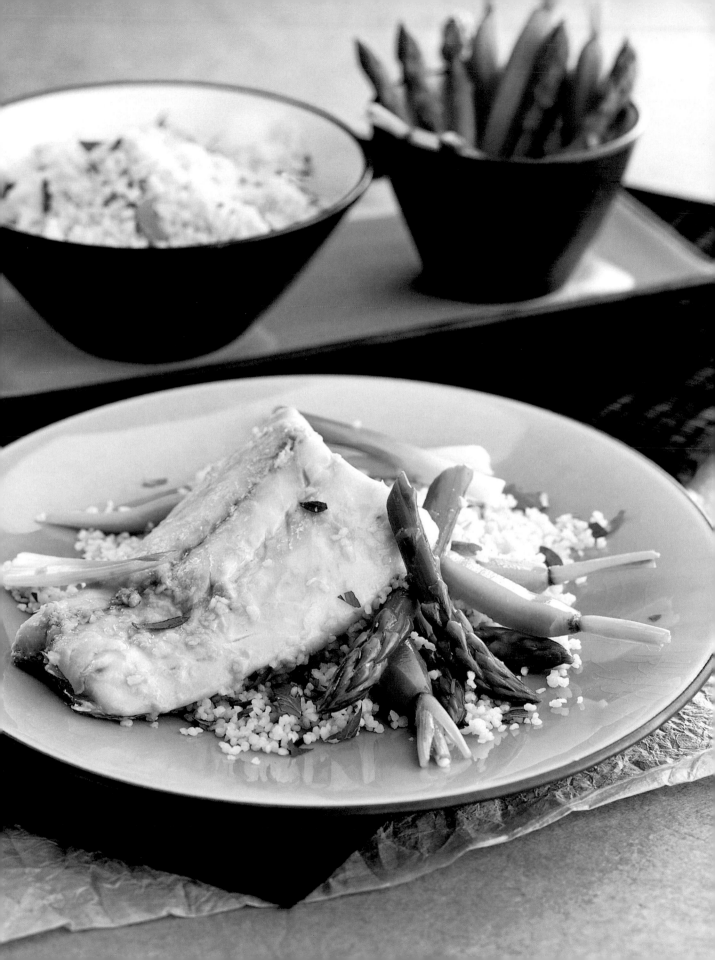

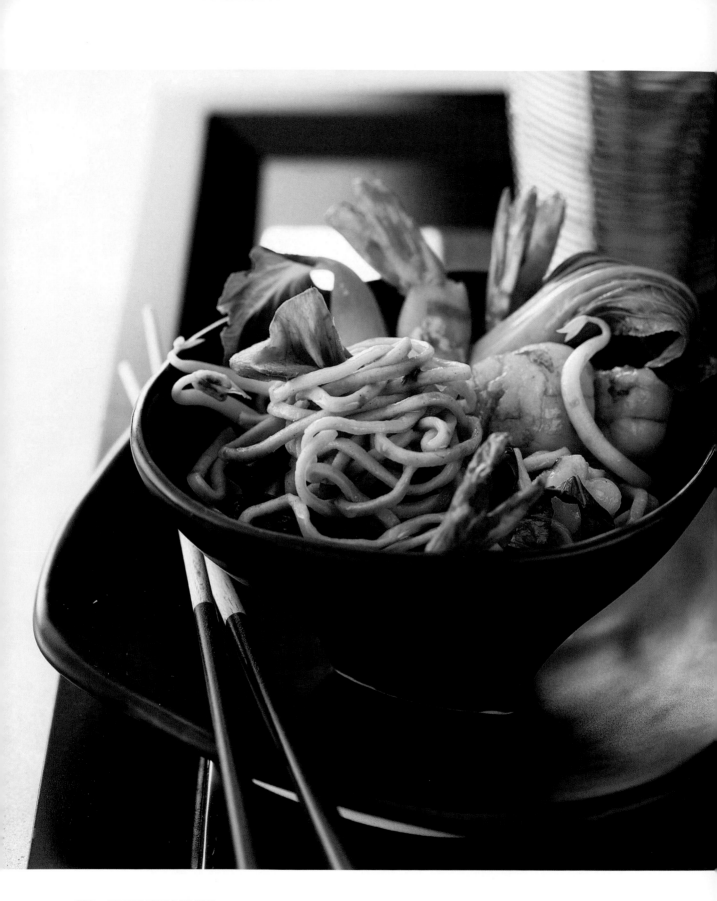

stir-fried scallops & *shrimp*

For a quick and delicious meal, this Asian seafood stir-fry is hard to beat. It requires very little oil, and the seaweed and vegetables add lots of flavor and texture. Pickled ginger is readily available in larger supermarkets.

SERVES 4   PREPARATION 15 MINUTES, PLUS 10 MINUTES SOAKING   COOKING 5 MINUTES

1 tablespoon (5 g) dried wakame seaweed

$1^1/_3$ cups (350 g) fresh thin egg noodles

juice of 1 lemon or 1 lime

2 teaspoons (10 ml) honey

1 tablespoon (15 ml) low-sodium soy sauce

4 scallops, about $^1/_2$ pound (200 g) total, quartered

24 peeled raw shrimp, about 6 ounces (170 g) total, tails left on if desired

2 teaspoons (10 ml) sunflower oil

1 teaspoon (5 ml) sesame oil

5 ounces (150 g) bok choy, leaves separated

$3^1/_3$ cups (300 g) bean sprouts, trimmed

3 teaspoons (15 ml) pickled ginger

Food Fact

WAKAME is usually sold dried and is rehydrated with water before using. It contains essential minerals, such as calcium, phosphorus, magnesium and iodine.

1 Put the wakame in a bowl, cover with $1^1/_4$ cups (300 ml) cold water and leave for 8–10 minutes to rehydrate; drain well. Put the noodles in a large bowl and add enough boiling water to cover them generously. Let soak for 4 minutes, or according to the package instructions, until tender. Drain when they are ready.

2 Meanwhile, combine the lemon juice, honey and half of the soy sauce. Pour the marinade over the scallops and shrimp and set aside to marinate for 5 minutes.

3 Drain the scallops and shrimp, reserving the marinade, and pat dry with paper towels. Heat a wok or heavy-bottom frying pan over medium–high heat, add the combined sunflower and sesame oils and swirl to coat the wok. Add the scallops and shrimp and stir-fry for 2–3 minutes, or until the shrimp have just turned pink and the scallops are opaque. Remove from the wok and set aside.

4 Add the bok choy, bean sprouts, reserved marinade, remaining soy sauce and the pickled ginger to the wok and stir-fry for 1–2 minutes.

5 Return the scallops and shrimp to the wok, add the wakame and stir-fry for 1 minute, or until just heated through. Serve with the egg noodles.

Each serving provides
369 calories, 26 g protein, 6 g fat (1 g saturated fat),
53 g carbohydrate (5 g sugars), 5 g fiber, 436 mg sodium

stir-fried squid with chile & fresh ginger

SERVES 4   PREPARATION 15 MINUTES
COOKING 10 MINUTES

1½ cups (300 g) basmati rice
2 tablespoons (30 ml) sunflower oil
2 red chilies, seeded and thinly sliced
2 cloves garlic, crushed
1 tablespoon (15 ml) finely grated
   fresh ginger
1 orange pepper, seeded and diced
1 cup (200 g) baby corn, halved
   diagonally
1 cup (200 g) small broccoli florets,
   halved
1 pound (500 g) fresh calamari
   (squid) rings
2 tablespoons (30 ml) low-sodium
   soy sauce
10 scallions, thinly sliced

1 Bring a large saucepan of water to a
  boil, add rice and cook until tender.
2 Heat the oil in a wok or heavy-bottom
  frying pan over medium heat and
  stir-fry chilies, garlic and ginger for
  2 minutes. Add the pepper, corn and
  broccoli and stir-fry for 3–4 minutes,
  or until the broccoli is almost tender.
3 Add the squid and stir-fry for 1–2
  minutes, or until just opaque. Add
  soy sauce and 2 tablespoons (30 ml)
  water and scatter scallions over all.
  Cook until bubbling and serve
  immediately with the rice.

Each serving provides
511 calories, 31 g protein, 12 g fat
(2 g saturated fat), 64 g carbohydrate
(3 g sugars), 5 g fiber, 439 mg sodium

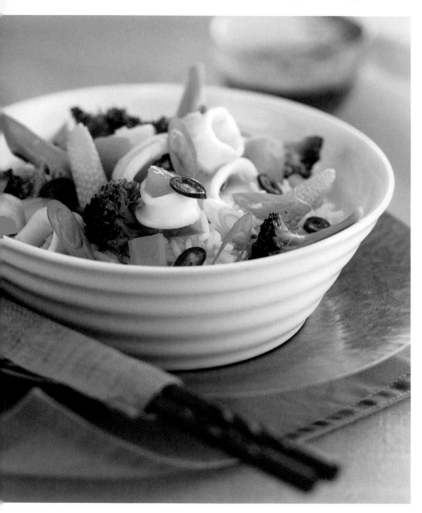

SQUID, or calamari, is an excellent source of low-fat protein and vitamin B$_{12}$.

BROCCOLI is an excellent source of beta-carotene, vitamin C and vitamin E —all powerful antioxidants that help to protect the body's cells against the damaging effects of free radicals.

scallops with noodle stir-fry & watercress

SERVES 4 PREPARATION 15 MINUTES
COOKING 10 MINUTES

1 cup (200 g) dried thin
  egg noodles
$^2/_3$ pound (300 g) scallops
1 clove garlic, crushed
grated zest of 1 lemon
1 teaspoon (5 ml) English mustard
4 sprigs fresh tarragon
3 tablespoons (45 ml) olive oil
$2^1/_2$ cups (600 g) ready-to-use stir-fry
  vegetables, such as broccoli,
  peppers, zucchini and cabbage
$^2/_3$ cup (150 g) watercress, trimmed

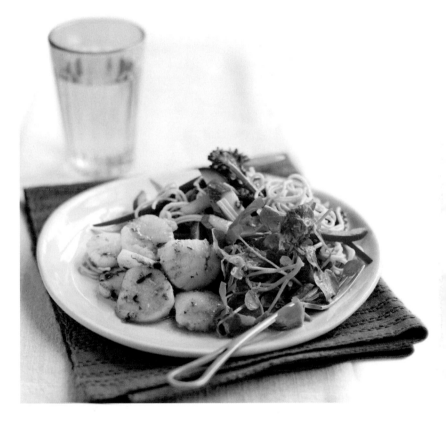

1 Put the noodles in a large heatproof bowl and cover generously with boiling water. Cover and set aside for 5 minutes, or until softened.

2 Cut the scallops in half widthwise and put into a bowl. Add the garlic, lemon zest, mustard, tarragon and 2 tablespoons (30 ml) of the oil. Mix well and set aside.

3 Heat the remaining oil in a wok or large frying pan over medium heat, add the vegetables and stir-fry for 5 minutes.

4 Drain the noodles, wipe the bowl with paper towels and return the noodles to the warm bowl. Add the vegetables and mix well. Set aside.

5 Add the scallops to the wok, along with all the marinade, and cook for 2–3 minutes, turning the scallops once, then remove from the wok.

Divide the vegetable and noodle mixture among four large plates, and arrange the scallops and watercress on the plates.

6 Add $^1/_3$ cup (75 ml) water to the wok and bring to a boil, stirring to loosen all the browned bits. Boil hard for a few seconds and spoon the boiling juices over the watercress to wilt it slightly. Serve immediately.

Each serving provides
412 calories, 19 g protein, 16 g fat (2 g saturated fat),
46 g carbohydrate (5 g sugars), 7 g fiber, 198 mg sodium

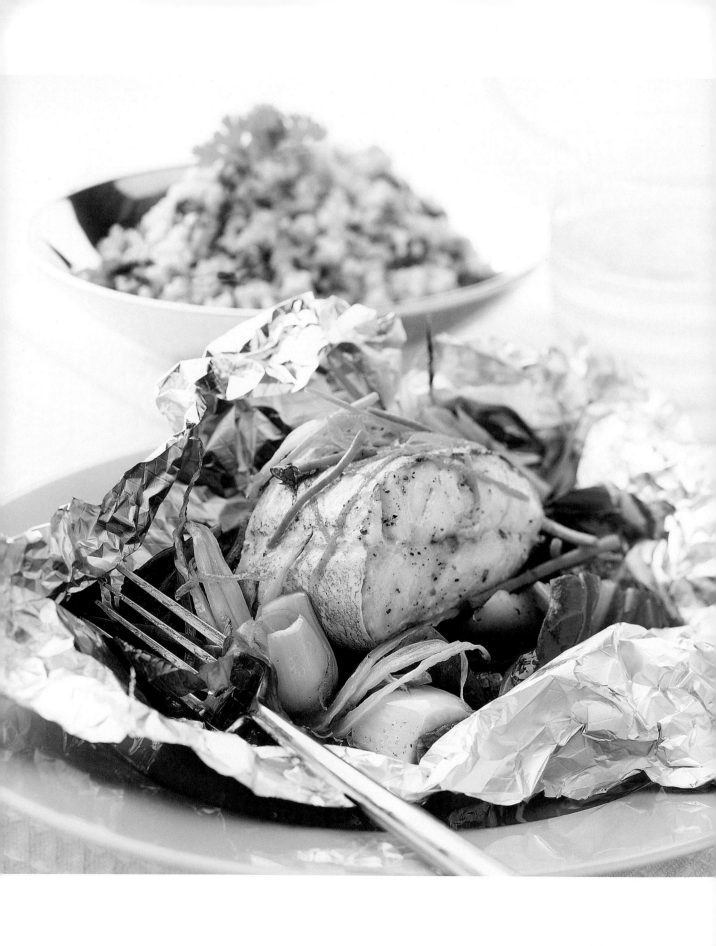

baked fish parcels

Lay a piece of fish on a bed of greens, season it with a few aromatics
and wrap it up tightly in a parcel and you have a simple, easy way
to cook fish—and seal in all the nutrients, too.

SERVES 4   PREPARATION 20 MINUTES   COOKING 15 MINUTES

1¼ cups (280 g) mixed Asian greens,
   such as bok choy and Chinese
   cabbage, chopped
4 fish steaks, such as halibut
   or haddock, about 5 ounces
   (140 g) each
grated zest and juice of
   ½ small orange
3 tablespoons (45 ml) shredded
   fresh basil
2 garlic cloves, finely chopped
½ cup (125 ml) dry white wine
1 tablespoon (15 ml) olive oil
½ bulb fennel, very thinly sliced
1 carrot, cut into thin strips
freshly ground black pepper

Bulgur and herb pilaf
1 cup (200 g) bulgur
1 tablespoon (15 ml) olive oil
juice of ½ lemon
1 garlic clove, finely chopped
2 tablespoons (30 ml) shredded
   fresh basil
2 tablespoons (30 ml) chopped
   fresh cilantro leaves
3 scallions, thinly sliced

1 Preheat the oven to 465°F (240°C). Cut four 12 inch
(30 cm) squares of foil or parchment paper. Arrange
one-quarter of the chopped Asian greens in the middle
of each square. Top with a piece of fish and cover with
orange zest and juice, basil, garlic, wine, oil, fennel and
carrot. Season to taste with pepper. Fold the foil over
to form a parcel, leaving a little air inside so the
ingredients can steam; twist the edges to seal. Place
the parcels on a baking sheet. Set aside.

2 To make the bulgur and herb pilaf, combine the bulgur
with 3¾ cups (900 ml) water in a large saucepan and
bring to a boil. Reduce heat to medium–low, cover and
cook for 12–15 minutes, or until just tender. Drain the
bulgur if necessary.

3 While the bulgur is cooking, put the fish parcels into the
oven and bake for 10 minutes. Open one of the parcels
to check that the fish is cooked; it will flake easily when
tested with a fork.

4 Fluff the bulgur with a fork and mix in the oil, lemon
juice, garlic, basil, cilantro and scallions. Season to
taste with pepper. Serve one fish parcel to each person,
and let them open it at the table (take care as steam is
hot). Serve the bulgur pilaf separately in a bowl.

OTHER IDEAS
+ *Cod or tuna can be used instead of halibut or haddock.*
+ *Replace the white wine with orange juice.*

Each serving provides
396 calories, 31 g protein, 11 g fat (2 g saturated fat),
34 g carbohydrate (4 g sugars), 9 g fiber, 167 mg sodium

roasted salmon with green beans

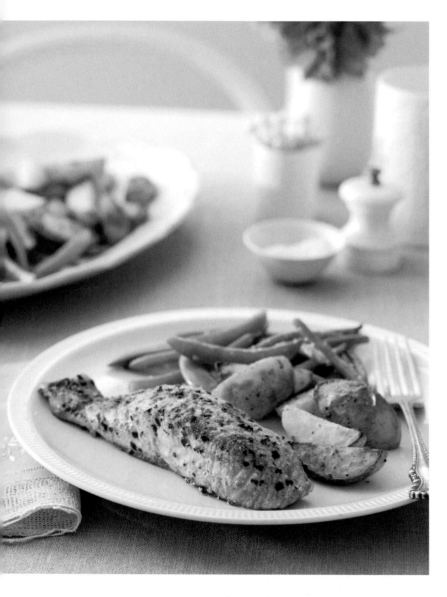

SERVES 4   PREPARATION 15 MINUTES
COOKING 15 MINUTES

1¹/₂ pounds (750 g) small new
   potatoes, scrubbed
2 tablespoons (30 ml) olive oil
pinch of salt and freshly ground
   black pepper
1 tablespoon (15 ml) piri piri spice mix
   (available from specialty food stores)
4 salmon fillets, about 5 ounces (150 g)
   each, skin removed
5 ounces (150 g) green beans, trimmed
5 ounces (150 g) sugar snap peas

1 Preheat the oven to 425°F (220°C).
   Line two baking pans with
   parchment paper.
2 Cut the potatoes lengthwise into
   wedges and toss them in a large bowl.
   with 1 tablespoon (15 ml) of oil; season
   with salt and pepper. Put the potatoes
   in a single layer on one of the pans.
   Rub the spice mix evenly over each
   side of the salmon fillets. Place them
   on the other pan; drizzle each portion
   with ¹/₂ teaspoon (2 ml) oil. Roast
   potatoes for 15 minutes, roast the
   salmon filets for 8–10 minutes,
   depending on their thickness.
3 While the fish is roasting, bring a
   saucepan of water to a boil. Add
   the beans and sugar snaps and cook
   over a medium–high heat for
   2–3 minutes, or until just tender.
   Drain and season with pepper.
4 Serve the salmon with the potatoes,
   green beans and sugar snap peas.

Each serving provides
442 calories, 36 g protein, 20 g fat
(4 g saturated fat), 29 g carbohydrate
(3 g sugars), 6 g fiber, 226 mg sodium

mediterranean *seafood pie*

SERVES 4 PREPARATION 10 MINUTES
COOKING 25 MINUTES

2 pounds (1 kg) potatoes
1$^1\!/_2$ tablespoons (22 ml) olive oil
1 large leek, white part only,
   thinly sliced
1 clove garlic, crushed
14$^1\!/_2$ ounce (400 ml) can
   diced tomatoes
$^1\!/_4$ teaspoon (1 ml) dried oregano
$^2\!/_3$ pound (350 g) frozen cooked
   mixed seafood, including
   mussels, shrimp and squid
freshly ground black pepper
$^1\!/_4$ cup (25 g) grated Parmesan

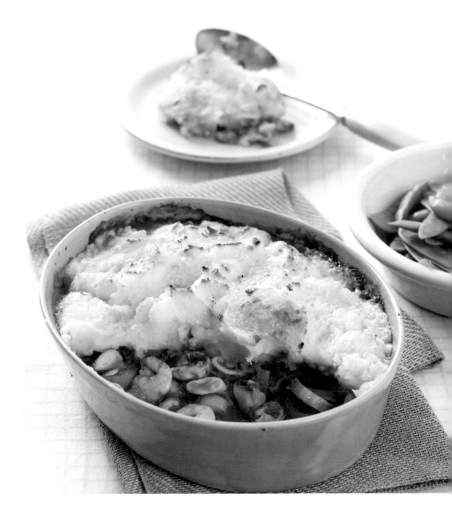

1 Peel the potatoes and cut into 1–2
   inch (3–5 cm) chunks. Bring a
   saucepan of water to a boil, add the
   potatoes and return to a boil.
   Simmer 10 minutes, or until tender.

2 Meanwhile, preheat the broiler to
   high. Heat the oil in a large
   saucepan over a medium–high heat
   and cook the leek and garlic for 2–3
   minutes, stirring, until the leek has
   softened. Add the tomatoes, rinsing
   out the can with 1 tablespoon
   (15 ml) water. Add the oregano and
   bring to a boil. Reduce the heat,
   cover and simmer for 2 minutes.

3 Add the seafood to the pan and
   return to a boil. Stir, cover the pan
   and simmer for another 2 minutes,
   or until seafood is thoroughly heated
   through. Season with pepper. Pour
   the seafood mixture into a 6-cup
   (1.5 liter) ovenproof dish.

4 Drain the potatoes, mash them and
   spoon them evenly over the top of the
   seafood, forking them up to the edge of
   the dish. Sprinkle with the Parmesan
   and broil for 12–13 minutes, or until
   the topping is golden.

Each serving provides
375 calories, 28 g protein, 12 g fat
(3 g saturated fat), 38 g carbohydrate
(5 g sugars), 6 g fiber, 342 mg sodium

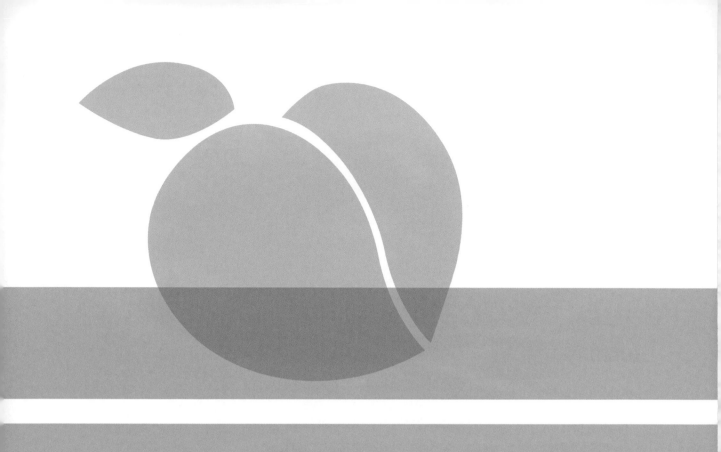

desserts & sweets

chapter 5

lemon mousse with strawberries

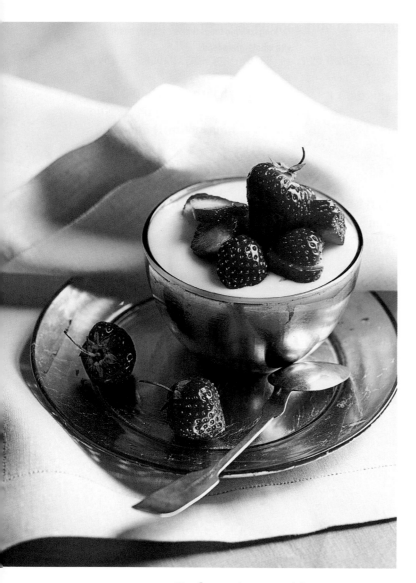

SERVES 8   PREPARATION 20 MINUTES, PLUS
3 HOURS CHILLING   COOKING 5 MINUTES

1 cup (250 g) strawberries, hulled and
  sliced thickly
2 teaspoons (10 ml) powdered gelatin
$^3/_4$ cup (165 g) sugar
2 teaspoons (10 ml) finely grated
  lemon zest
$^1/_2$ cup (125 ml) freshly squeezed
  lemon juice
1 tablespoon (15 ml) extra light olive oil
1 large egg
$1^1/_3$ cups (340 ml) fat-free plain yogurt

1 Put 3 tablespoons (45 ml) cold water in
  a small bowl. Sprinkle gelatin evenly
  over the water; let soften for 5 minutes.
2 Put another 3 tablespoons (45 ml)
  water, the sugar, lemon zest, lemon
  juice, oil and egg in a saucepan and
  whisk together until well combined.
  Place the pan over a low heat and
  cook, whisking constantly, for about
  5 minutes, or until the mixture is hot.
  Whisk in the softened gelatin and
  cook, whisking constantly, until the
  gelatin has dissolved.
3 Remove from the heat, transfer the
  lemon mixture to a bowl and cool to
  room temperature, whisking
  occasionally. Whisk in the yogurt.
4 Layer the strawberries and lemon
  mousse into eight dessert bowls and
  place in the fridge to chill for about
  3 hours, or until set.

Each serving provides
148 calories, 5 g protein, 3 g fat
(1 g saturated fat), 26 g carbohydrate
(25 g sugars), 1 g fiber, 52 mg sodium

fresh berries *with sabayon sauce*

SERVES 4   PREPARATION 10 MINUTES
COOKING 15 MINUTES

1 cup (250 g) strawberries or
   blueberries
1 cup (125 g) raspberries
3 egg yolks
⅓ cup (80 g) superfine sugar
½ cup (125 ml) brandy, rum or
   orange-flavored liqueur

1 Hull the strawberries, and divide
   the strawberries and raspberries
   among four dessert glasses.
2 Put the egg yolks and sugar in a
   heatproof bowl and whisk to
   combine. Place the bowl over a
   saucepan of gently simmering
   water (or use a double boiler) and
   cook gently, whisking constantly,
   for 2–3 minutes, or until warm
   and creamy.
3 Whisking continuously, add the
   brandy in a thin steady stream,
   and continue to whisk for another
   10–12 minutes, or until the sauce is
   thick. Remove from the heat.
4 Spoon the sabayon sauce over the
   berries and serve immediately.
   You can serve this dessert on its
   own, or accompany it with crisp
   dessert biscuits.

Each serving provides
211 calories, 3 g protein, 4 g fat
(1 g saturated fat), 24 g carbohydrate
(24 g sugars), 3 g fiber, 11 mg sodium

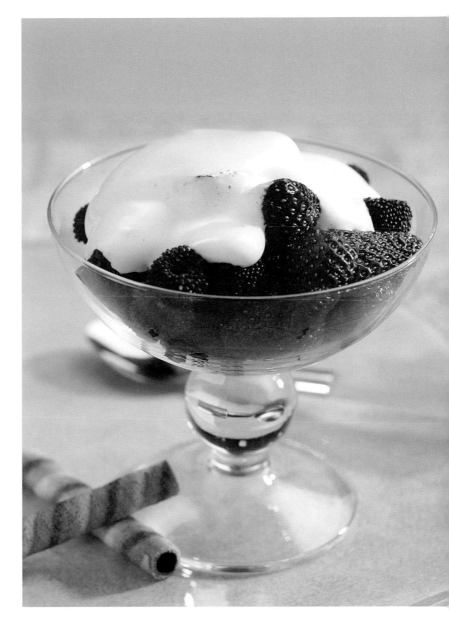

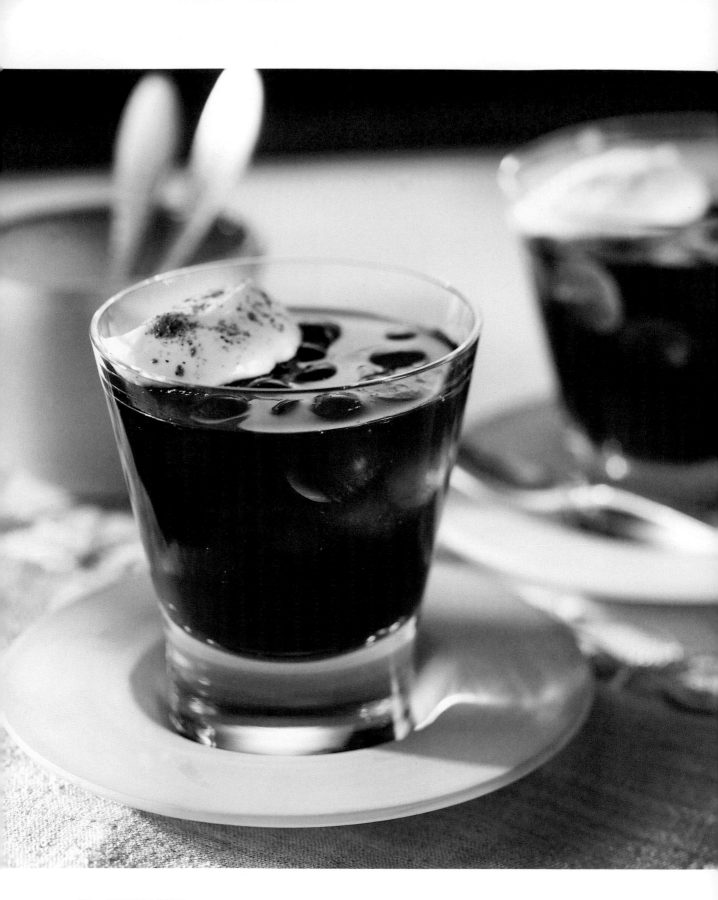

mulled *grape jelly*

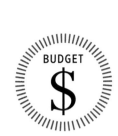

BUDGET
$

Jellies are not just for kids. This sophisticated version is made using a refreshing spiced wine, which becomes a jelly studded with fresh grapes. These jellies satisfy a sweet tooth and are virtually fat free—and they definitely look lovely served in a sparkling glass dish or wine glass.

SERVES 4   PREPARATION 10 MINUTES, PLUS CHILLING AND 4 HOURS SETTING   COOKING 10 MINUTES

1 cup (250 g) seedless red
  or black grapes
½ small orange
1 cup (250 ml) red wine
2 star anise
2 tablespoons (30 ml) superfine sugar
2 teaspoons (10 ml) powdered gelatin
1 cup (250 ml) red grape juice
Greek-style yogurt, to serve
pinch of freshly grated nutmeg,
  to serve

1 Leave the grapes whole or cut them in half if large, and divide among four large glass tumblers or dishes. Put in the fridge to chill.

2 Meanwhile, make the jelly. Thinly slice a long strip of zest from the orange half, squeeze the juice from the orange and set aside. Place the zest in a saucepan with the wine and star anise. Heat gently until almost boiling, reduce the heat, cover and simmer for 10 minutes. Remove the pan from the heat, add the sugar and stir until it has dissolved.

3 Strain the sweetened wine into a bowl. Sprinkle the gelatin over the surface and stir gently until dissolved. Add the reserved orange juice and the grape juice and set aside to cool for 5 minutes, or until the liquid is lukewarm.

4 Pour the jelly mixture over the grapes in the glasses and set aside until completely cool, then transfer to the fridge for 4 hours, or until set.

5 Serve each jelly topped with a little yogurt and sprinkled with nutmeg.

Each serving provides
176 calories, 3 g protein, 1 g fat (<1 g saturated fat),
29 g carbohydrate (27 g sugars), 1 g fiber, 25 mg sodium

coconut-topped sweet potato pudding

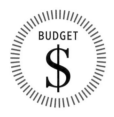

BUDGET
$

Sweet potatoes come in various skin and flesh colors, from cream to purple to pinky-orange, and their use is not limited to savory dishes. The orange variety is used here for its intense sweetness and moist flesh, which goes well with spices such as ginger, cinnamon and nutmeg.

SERVES 10   PREPARATION 15 MINUTES   COOKING 2 HOURS

2 teaspoons (10 ml) vegetable oil
2 orange sweet potatoes, about
    1 pound (500 g), peeled, grated
1 1/2 cups (375 ml) light
    evaporated milk
1 tablespoon (15 ml) vegetable oil
1/2 cup (115 g) firmly packed soft
    brown sugar
2 tablespoons (30 ml) orange juice
    concentrate
1/2 teaspoon (2 ml) ground ginger
1/2 teaspoon (2 ml) ground cloves
1/2 teaspoon (2 ml) ground allspice
pinch of salt
1 large egg, lightly beaten
4 large egg whites, lightly beaten
1/2 cup (30 g) shaved coconut

1 Preheat the oven to 350°F (180°C). Lightly grease an 8 cup (2 liter) baking dish with the oil.
2 Combine all the ingredients except the coconut in a large bowl. Pour the sweet potato mixture into the baking dish and cover with foil.
3 Bake for 1 hour. Top with the coconut and bake for another 10 minutes, or until the center is set and the coconut turns golden.

Each serving provides
178 calories, 7 g protein, 6 g fat (3 g saturated fat), 25 g carbohydrate (20 g sugars), 1 g fiber, 137 mg sodium

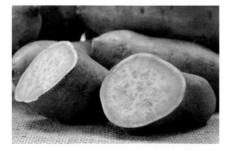

Superfood
SWEET POTATOES are an excellent source of beta-carotene, fiber and vitamins C and A. They are particularly recommended for people with diabetes because they have a low glycemic index.

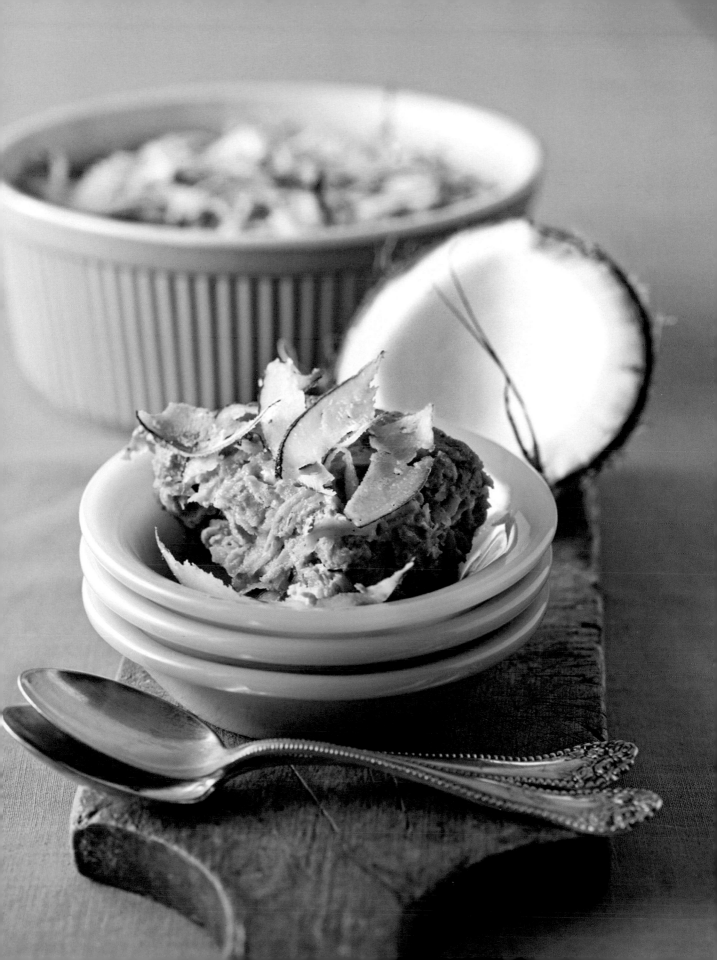

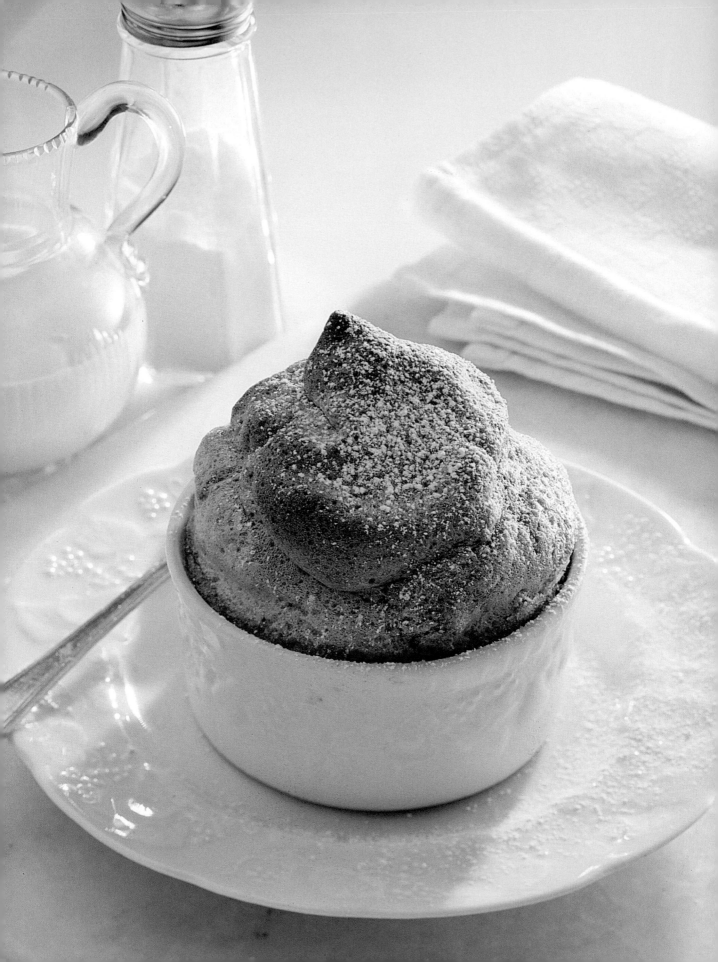

hot raspberry *soufflés*

Soufflés make an impressive dinner party finale and aren't as difficult to make as you might think. Once cooked, they must be eaten straight from the oven to capture the light, melt-in-your-mouth texture. These hot soufflés are made with raspberries, giving them a beautiful color as well as fruity flavor.

SERVES 4   PREPARATION 25 MINUTES   COOKING 15 MINUTES

2 teaspoons (10 ml) unsalted butter,
   at room temperature
$^1/_3$ cup (100 g) superfine sugar
1 cup (250 g) raspberries
1 tablespoon (15 ml) kirsch or
   cherry liqueur (optional)
4 large egg whites
2 teaspoons (10 ml)
   confectioners' sugar
cream, to serve (optional)

1 Before you sit down to your main course, preheat the oven to 375°F (190°C). Grease the insides of four 1 cup (250 ml) soufflé dishes or ramekins with butter, and coat evenly with some of the superfine sugar, tapping out the excess. Place the dishes on a baking sheet.

2 Purée the raspberries by pressing the fruit through a sieve, using the back of a spoon. Stir the kirsch, if using, into the purée.

3 When you have finished the main course, whisk the egg whites with an electric mixer until stiff but not dry, and gradually whisk in the remaining superfine sugar. Beat until the mixture is shiny.

4 Using a large metal spoon, carefully fold the raspberry purée into the egg whites, and spoon the mixture into the dishes and make a swirl on top of each. Leaving space above for the soufflés to rise, cook in the center of the oven for 12–14 minutes, or until well risen and lightly set.

5 Remove the soufflés from the oven and sift the confectioners' sugar over the top of each. If you like, serve drizzled with a little cream.

Each serving provides
180 calories, 4 g protein, 2 g fat (1 g saturated fat),
32 g carbohydrate (30 g sugars), 3 g fiber, 56 mg sodium

raspberry & passion fruit
sponge roll

This light, almost fat-free sponge cake, rolled up around a crushed raspberry and passion fruit filling, makes a very delicious dessert. It's ideal for late summer, when red ripe raspberries are at their sweetest.

SERVES 8   PREPARATION 20 MINUTES   COOKING 10 MINUTES

2³/₄ cups (340 g) raspberries,
   plus extra to serve
¹/₄ cup (30 g) confectioners'
   sugar, sifted
4 passion fruit, halved
a few sprigs fresh mint, to garnish

Sponge
3 large eggs
¹/₂ cup (115 g) raw superfine sugar
³/₄ cup (110 g) all-purpose flour
1 tablespoon (15 ml) tepid water

1 Put half of the raspberries into a bowl with the confectioners' sugar and crush lightly with a fork. Scoop out the passion fruit pulp and stir into the raspberries.
2 Preheat the oven to 400°F (200°C). Grease a 9 x 13 inch (23 x 33 cm) Swiss roll pan and line the bottom with parchment paper.

3 To make the sponge, put the eggs and sugar in a large bowl and beat with an electric mixer until very thick and pale, and the mixture leaves a trail on the surface when the beaters are lifted out.
4 Sift half of the flour over the mixture and gently fold it in with a large metal spoon. Sift over the remaining flour and fold in together with the tepid water.
5 Pour the mixture into the prepared pan and shake gently to fill the corners. Bake for 10–12 minutes, or until the sponge is golden and springs back when pressed gently.
6 Turn out onto a sheet of parchment paper that is slightly larger than the sponge. Peel off the lining paper. Trim the crusty edges of the sponge.
7 Spread the crushed raspberry mixture over the hot sponge, leaving a ¹/₂ inch (1 cm) border. Scatter the reserved raspberries over the sponge. Carefully roll up the sponge from one of the short edges and place, seam side down, on a serving plate. Garnish with a few extra raspberries and the mint sprigs and serve warm or cold, cut into slices.

Each serving provides
171 calories, 5 g protein, 3 g fat (1 g saturated fat), 31 g carbohydrate (21 g sugars), 4 g fiber, 32 mg sodium

BERRIES are bursting with vitamin C, and are rich in dietary fiber. They are also an excellent source of immune-enhancing antioxidants.

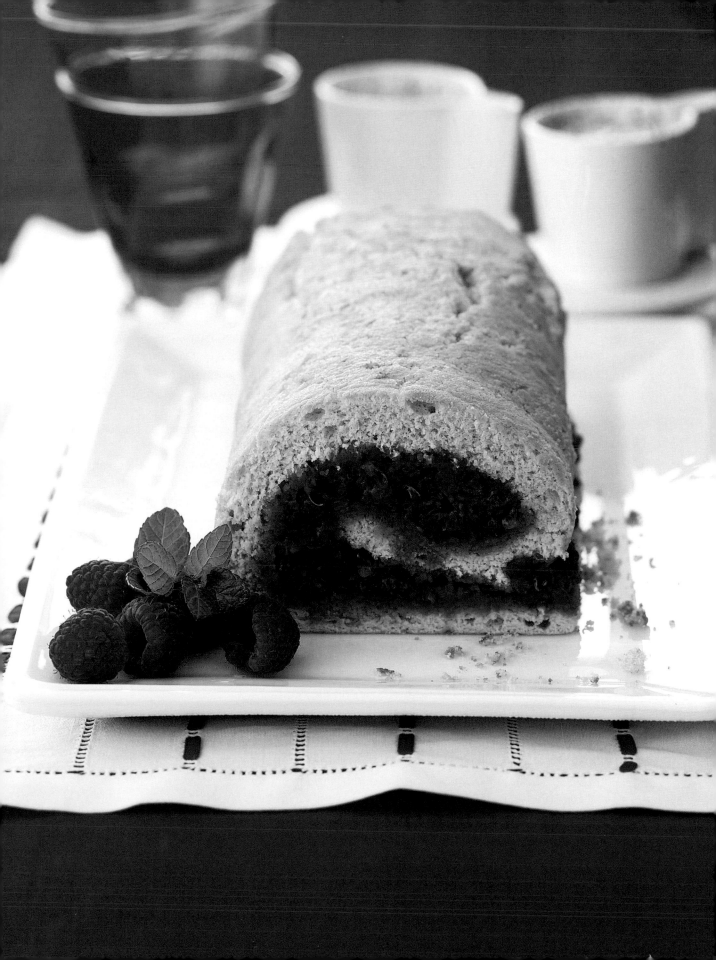

old-fashioned secret-ingredient *chocolate cake*

Shhhh . . . don't let on that the secret in this delectable to-die-for cake is actually tomato juice, which adds surprising richness and moisture to the batter.

SERVES 16   PREPARATION 15 MINUTES   COOKING 30 MINUTES

$^3/_4$ cup (175 ml) tomato juice

$^1/_4$ cup (50 ml) water

$^2/_3$ cup (150 g) unsweetened cocoa powder

$2^1/_4$ cups (550 g) all-purpose flour

1 teaspoon (5 ml) baking soda

$^1/_2$ teaspoon (2 ml) baking powder

$^1/_4$ teaspoon (1 ml) salt

$1^1/_2$ cups (375 g) sugar

$^1/_2$ cup (125 ml) vegetable oil

3 large eggs

$1^1/_2$ teaspoons (7 ml) vanilla extract

Icing

1 ounce (25 g) unsweetened chocolate

2 tablespoons (30 ml) low-fat (1%) milk

1 tablespoon (15 ml) unsweetened cocoa powder

4 ounces (125 g) one-third-less-fat cream cheese

$2^1/_2$ cups (625 g) confectioner's sugar, sifted

$^1/_2$ cup (125 g) seedless raspberry jam

1 Preheat oven to 350°F (180°C). Coat two 9 inch (23 cm) round cake pans with nonstick cooking spray.

2 In small saucepan, bring tomato juice and water to a boil. Whisk in cocoa powder until smooth. Remove from heat.

3 In medium bowl, stir together flour, baking soda, baking powder, and salt.

4 In large bowl, beat together sugar, oil, eggs, and 1 teaspoon (5 ml) vanilla extract until combined. Beat in cocoa mixture. Beat in flour mixture just until evenly moistened. Divide batter between prepared pans.

5 Bake until toothpick inserted in centers of cakes comes out clean, 25 to 30 minutes. Transfer pans to wire rack. Let cool 10 minutes. Turn cakes out onto rack. Let cool completely.

6 Prepare icing: In medium microwave-safe bowl, microwave together chocolate and milk on high power 1 minute. Stir until smooth. Whisk in cocoa powder until smooth. Whisk in cream cheese and $^1/_2$ teaspoon (2 ml) vanilla extract. Stir in confectioner's sugar until combined.

7 Place one cake layer on flat plate or platter. Spread top of this layer with jam. Place remaining layer over layer with jam on it. Spread icing over sides and top of cake.

Each serving provides
350 calories, 5 g protein, 11 g fat (2.5 g saturated fat), 61 g carbohydrate (44 g sugars), 2 g fiber, 210 mg sodium

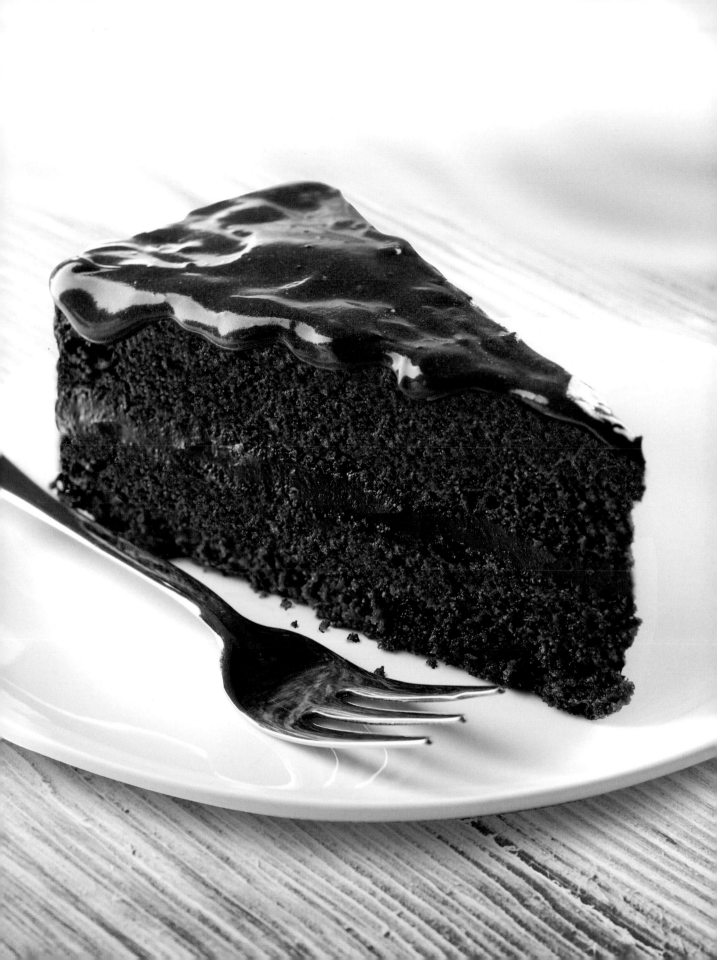

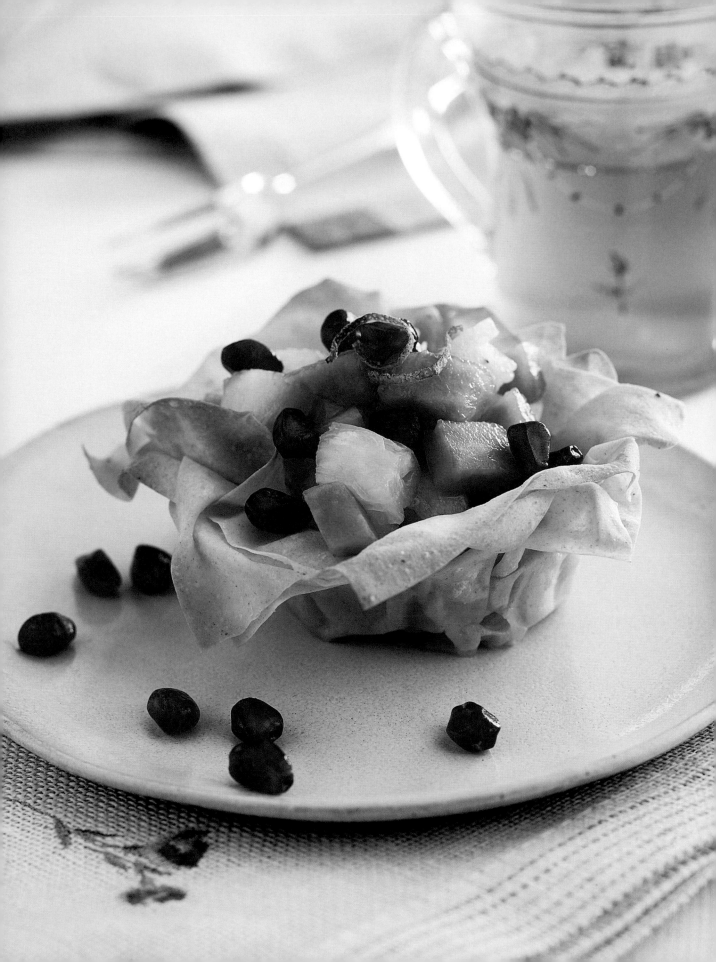

tropical *phyllo baskets*

This fruity dessert is made with sheets of phyllo, baked in a muffin pan to make crisp, petal-like baskets. They're filled with a creamy mango purée and topped with papaya, pineapple and pomegranate seeds.

SERVES 6   PREPARATION 35 MINUTES   COOKING 5 MINUTES

1 tablespoon (20 ml) unsalted
  butter, melted
3 sheets phyllo pastry, 12 x 20 inches
  (30 x 50 cm) each

Fruit filling
1 large mango
2 tablespoons (30 ml) reduced-fat
  fromage frais or Greek-style
  yogurt
1 papaya, cubed
1 small pineapple, cubed
seeds from 1 small pomegranate
finely grated zest of 1 lime

1 Preheat the oven to 375° (190°C). Using a little melted butter, lightly grease six cups of a standard muffin pan (or use individual muffin pans if you have them).

2 Lay the phyllo sheets on the work surface, one on top of the other. Cut the stack into 4 inch (12.5 cm) squares, trimming off the excess pastry. You will have 24 squares.

3 Line each muffin cup with one square of phyllo pastry and brush very lightly with melted butter. Place another square on top, with the corners offset, and brush with butter. Continue layering the phyllo squares in this way, using four sheets for each basket. Bake the phyllo baskets for 5–6 minutes, or until golden. Let cool.

4 To make the fruit filling, slice the mango flesh from the pit, chop into small chunks and put into a blender or food processor. Add the fromage frais and blend to form a smooth purée.

5 Shortly before serving, spoon the mango purée into the phyllo baskets. Top with the papaya and pineapple, then scatter with the pomegranate seeds and lime zest.

Each serving provides
156 calories, 4 g protein, 3 g fat (2 g saturated fat),
27 g carbohydrate (19 g sugars), 4 g fiber, 118 mg sodium

PAPAYA is a useful source of vitamin A, derived from its beta-carotene content. It also provides good amounts of vitamin C plus calcium, iron and zinc.

POMEGRANATE SEEDS are deliciously sweet–tart and crunchy, and provide some vitamin C and fiber.

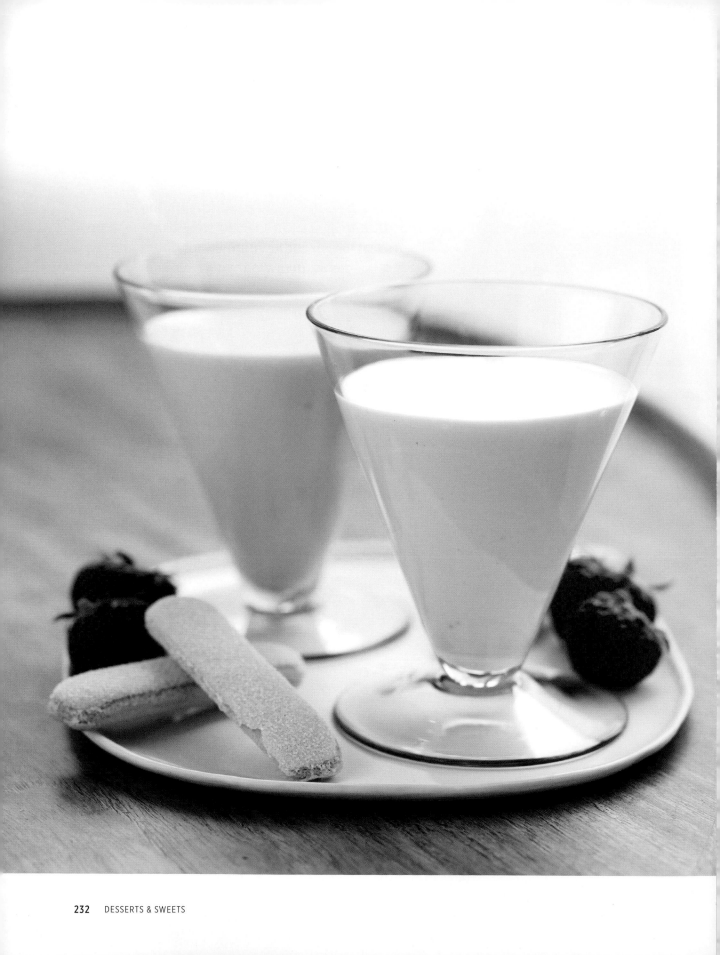

passion fruit & *honey zabaglione*

Zabaglione is a classic Italian dessert of egg yolks whisked over heat until thickened. The egg yolks are traditionally flavored with sweet Marsala dessert wine, but this fruity version uses passion fruit juice. It's extra delicious when scooped up with ladyfinger biscuits or strawberries.

SERVES 4   PREPARATION 10 MINUTES   COOKING 10 MINUTES

4 passion fruit
1 tablespoon (15 ml) boiling water
3 tablespoons (45 ml) honey
4 large egg yolks
2 teaspoons (10 ml) lemon juice

1 Cut each passion fruit in half and scoop the pulp and seeds into a sieve set over a large heatproof bowl. Sieve the fruit thoroughly, trickle the boiling water over the seed mixture in the sieve and scrape again with a spoon. Scrape any pulp from underneath the sieve into the bowl, too. Discard the seeds.

2 Half-fill a saucepan with boiling water and heat to a simmer. Put the honey, egg yolks and lemon juice into the bowl containing the passion fruit juice and beat well with an electric mixer. Set the bowl over the pan of barely simmering water and continue to whisk until the mixture is pale and thick and holds a trail when the beaters are lifted out. This takes about 10 minutes and the mixture will look like a slightly soft, sponge mixture when ready. Make sure the water is barely simmering. If you let it boil, the eggs will separate.

3 Remove the bowl from the pan and continue to whisk for another 1 minute. Spoon or pour the mixture into four glasses and serve immediately.

Each serving provides
130 calories, 3 g protein, 5 g fat (1 g saturated fat),
19 g carbohydrate (19 g sugars), 3 g fiber, 16 mg sodium

Serve the bowl of zabaglione as a dip, keeping it warm over a small saucepan of hot water at the table. Offer chunks of banana, strawberries, cherries, ladyfinger biscuits and biscotti to dip.

To make a classic zabaglione use 2 tablespoons (30 ml) superfine sugar and $^2/_3$ cup (150 ml) sweet Marsala instead of the passion fruit, honey and lemon juice.

mango cream in brandy-snap baskets

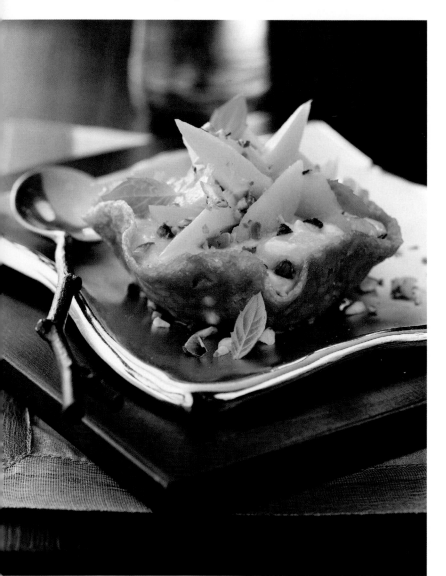

SERVES 6   PREPARATION 15 MINUTES
COOKING NONE

1 large mango
2 passion fruit
1 tablespoon (15 ml) good-quality lemon curd
1 teaspoon (5 ml) finely grated lemon zest
1 cup (200 ml) low-fat Greek-style yogurt
6 brandy-snap baskets (available at specialty food stores or online)
1 tablespoon (15 ml) chopped pistachios
fresh mint leaves, to garnish

1 Remove the flesh from the mango. Chop half, put in a food processor or blender and process to a smooth purée; put into a bowl. Chop the remaining mango flesh into smaller pieces and set aside.
2 Cut the passion fruit in half and scoop the seeds and pulp into the mango purée. Stir in the lemon curd, lemon zest and yogurt and fold together until well combined.
3 Spoon the fruit and yogurt cream into the brandy-snap baskets and top with the mango. Scatter a few chopped pistachios over the top of each serving and garnish with mint leaves. Serve immediately while the baskets are crisp.

Each serving provides
183 calories, 5 g protein, 7 g fat (2 g saturated fat), 25 g carbohydrate (20 g sugars), 2 g fiber, 60 mg sodium

date & orange salad

SERVES 4   PREPARATION 15 MINUTES, PLUS
1 HOUR CHILLING   COOKING 10 MINUTES

1 pinch of saffron threads
3 cardamom pods, bruised
1 inch (2.5 cm) strip lemon zest
1 tablespoon (15 ml) honey
1 teaspoon (5 ml) rosewater
3 large oranges, peeled, thickly sliced
8 fresh dates, pitted and quartered
2 tablespoons (30 ml) toasted
  pistachios, roughly chopped
2 tablespoons (30 ml) toasted
  slivered almonds

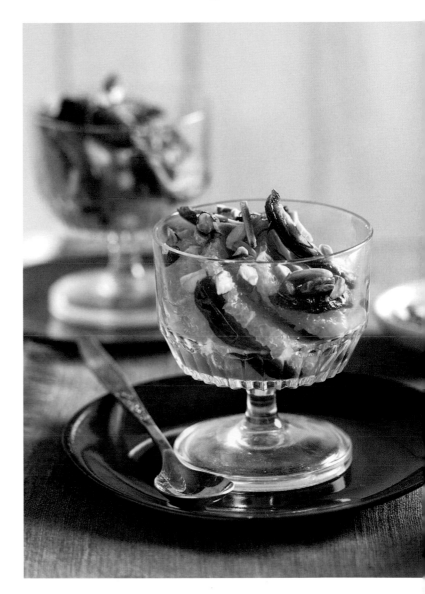

1 Combine $^1/_2$ cup (125 ml) water, the
  saffron threads, cardamom, strip of
  lemon zest and honey in a saucepan
  over medium heat. Stir until the
  mixture comes to a boil, reduce
  the heat to low and simmer for
  4–5 minutes, or until slightly
  thickened. Discard the zest. Stir
  in the rosewater and let cool.
2 Combine the oranges and dates in
  a serving bowl. Pour the rosewater
  syrup over the oranges, cover and
  refrigerate for 1 hour. Remove and
  discard the cardamom pods.
3 Sprinkle the salad with the pistachios
  and almonds and serve.

COOK'S TIP

+ *Bruise the cardamom pods by putting
  them on a chopping board and gently
  pressing down with the flat side of
  a knife blade until the pods flatten
  and open slightly at one end. This helps
  release the flavor of the cardamom.*

Each serving provides
179 calories, 4 g protein, 4 g fat
(<1 g saturated fat), 32 g carbohydrate
(30 g sugars), 6 g fiber, 9 mg sodium

rhubarb, ginger &
blueberry compote

SERVES 4   PREPARATION 5 MINUTES
COOKING 10 MINUTES, PLUS 30 MINUTES
CHILLING (OPTIONAL)

1¼ pounds (600 g) rhubarb
3 tablespoons (45 ml) sugar
¼ cup (50 g) crystallized ginger, cut
  into very thin slices
½ cup (125 g) blueberries

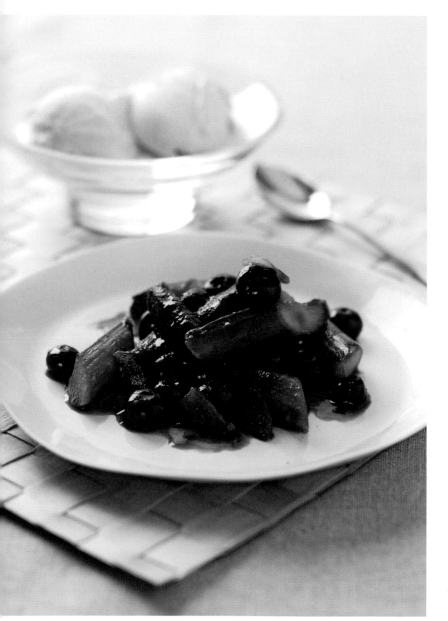

1 Cut the rhubarb into 1 inch
  (2.5 cm) lengths and place in a
  large saucepan. Sprinkle the
  sugar over the rhubarb and add
  1 tablespoon (15 ml) water. Cook
  over high heat for 30 seconds, or
  until the sugar begins to dissolve.
2 Reduce the heat to medium or
  medium–low, so that the rhubarb
  simmers. Cover the pan and
  simmer for 5–8 minutes, stirring
  once, until the rhubarb is tender
  but not mushy.
3 Remove the pan from the heat,
  add the crystallized ginger slices
  and blueberries and stir gently
  to combine. Serve warm, or chill
  for 30 minutes before serving.

COOK'S TIP

+ *Small, fresh stalks of rhubarb are
  usually tender and need just the
  ends of the stalks trimmed and the
  poisonous leaves discarded. Larger
  or older stalks should be thinly
  peeled to remove the skin, which
  can be stringy.*

Each serving provides
124 calories, 2 g protein, <1 g fat
(0 g saturated fat), 26 g carbohydrate
(25 g sugars), 4 g fiber, 20 mg sodium

berry & *passion fruit salad*

SERVES 6 PREPARATION 15 MINUTES
COOKING NONE

3 cups (450 g) strawberries, halved
1¼ cups (155 g) raspberries
¾ cup (100 g) blackberries
⅔ cup (100 g) blueberries
⅔ cup (100 g) mixed red currants
   and black currants, stalks removed
2 passion fruit
1 tablespoon (15 ml) superfine sugar
juice of ½ lemon or lime

1 Mix the strawberries, raspberries,
   blackberries, blueberries, red
   currants and black currants
   together in a bowl.
2 Cut each passion fruit in half and
   scoop the pulp and seeds into
   a sieve set over the bowl of berries.
   Using the back of a spoon, rub the
   pulp and seeds firmly to press all
   the juice through the sieve on the
   berries. Reserve a few of the seeds
   in the sieve and discard the rest.
3 Add the sugar and lemon juice to
   the berries. Gently toss together.
   Sprinkle the reserved passion fruit
   seeds over the top. Serve or cover
   and chill briefly.

Each serving provides
61 calories, 2 g protein, <1 g fat
(0 g saturated fat), 11 g carbohydrate
(11 g sugars), 6 g fiber, 7 mg sodium

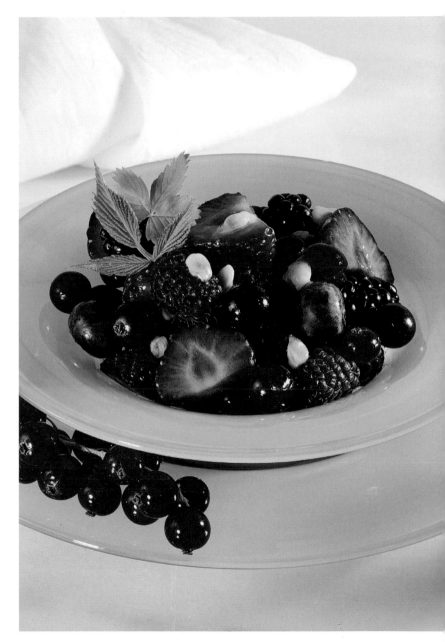

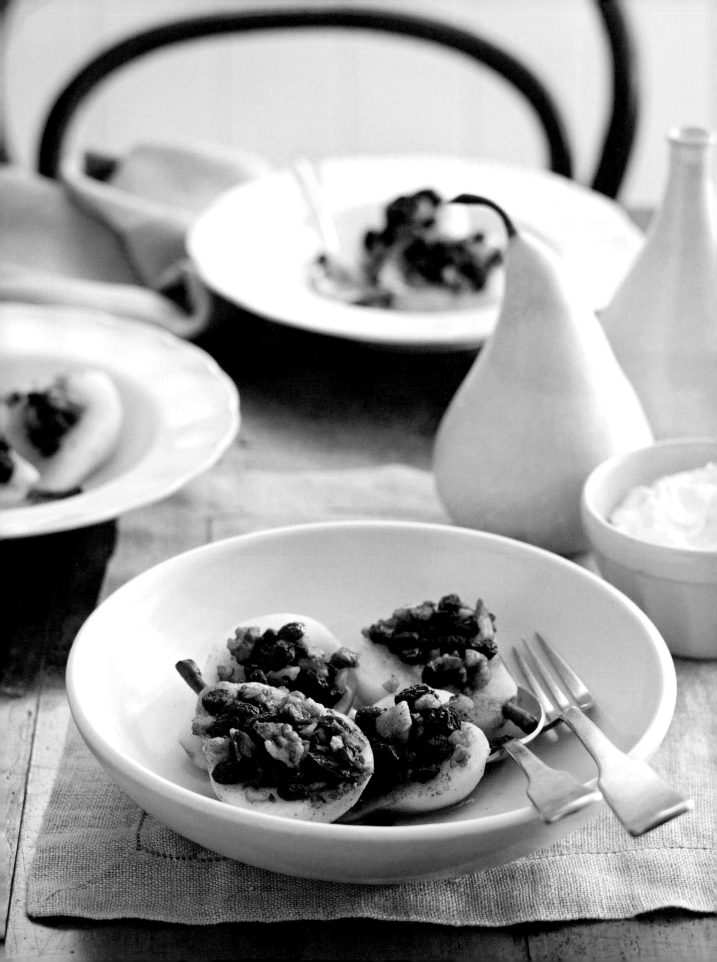

pears with *walnuts & raisins*

Everyone loves a simple poached pear dessert—and this one, made with fresh pears topped with walnuts and raisins, is a delicious and low-fat treat. To cut down on the long cooking time needed to render them soft, the pears are cooked in the microwave.

SERVES 4   PREPARATION 10 MINUTES   COOKING 10 MINUTES

4 small ripe pears
1/4 cup (50 g) raisins
2 tablespoons (30 ml) chopped
  walnuts
1/2 teaspoon (2 ml) ground cinnamon
1 tablespoon (15 ml) honey
low-fat plain yogurt, to serve

1 Peel the pears, cut them in half lengthwise and scoop out the cores. Place the pear halves in a shallow, round microwave-safe dish, with the wide ends of the pears touching the side of the dish.

2 Combine the raisins, walnuts and cinnamon in a bowl, and sprinkle evenly over the pears. Mix the honey with 2 teaspoons (10 ml) water and drizzle over the pears.

3 Cover the dish and microwave on medium–high for 8–12 minutes, or until the pears are tender. If you want to cook them in the oven, the pears will take 30–40 minutes in a 375°F (190°C) oven. Serve with the juices from the bottom of the dish drizzled over the pears, and add a dollop or two of yogurt.

Each serving provides
143 calories, 1 g protein, 3 g fat (<1 g saturated fat), 29 g carbohydrate (24 g sugars), 3 g fiber, 6 mg sodium

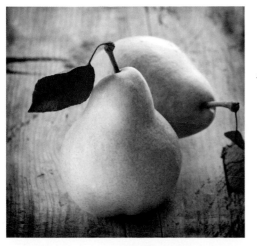

Food Fact
  PEARS make a great energy-boosting snack and are one of the most easily digested fruit. They provide potassium, copper, vitamin C and pectin, a type of soluble fiber, which helps to lower blood cholesterol levels and regulate blood-sugar levels. Eating pears with the skin left on significantly boosts the fiber content, as about half of the fiber is found in the skin.

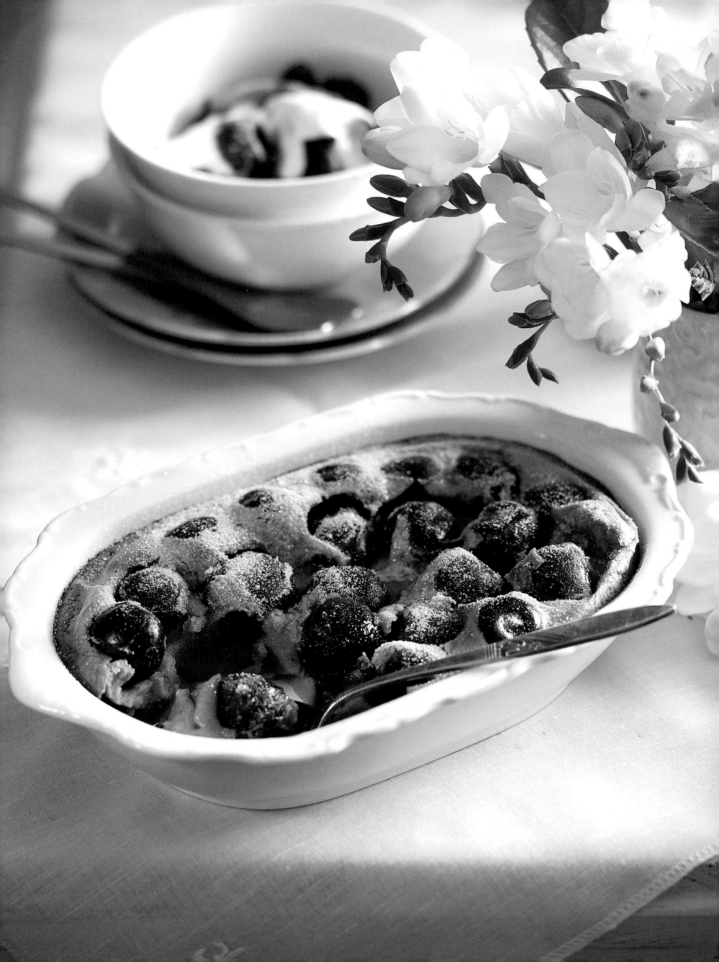

cherry clafoutis

Clafoutis is a classic French dessert in which fruit is baked in a sweetened batter. Typically fresh cherries are used, but this dessert would also work with fresh or canned plums, peaches or apricots.

SERVES 4   PREPARATION 15 MINUTES   COOKING 30 MINUTES

2 eggs
1/3 cup (50 g) all-purpose flour
1/2 teaspoon (2 ml) ground cinnamon
3/4 cup (180 ml) light evaporated milk
2 tablespoons (30 ml) honey
1 teaspoon (5 ml) vanilla extract
1 teaspoon (5 ml) reduced-fat canola spread
1 cup (200 g) fresh, canned or frozen pitted black cherries, thawed

2 teaspoons (10 ml) superfine sugar

1 Preheat the oven to 400°F (200°C). Whisk the eggs in a large bowl until smooth, and gradually beat in the flour and cinnamon. While beating continuously, add the evaporated milk, honey and vanilla. Continue beating until smooth.

2 Lightly grease a shallow 3 cup (750 ml) ovenproof dish with the canola spread, and set the dish on a baking tray. Spread the cherries in a single layer on the bottom of the prepared dish. Pour the batter over the cherries.

3 Bake for 20–30 minutes, or until cooked and well risen, and a skewer inserted in the center comes out clean. Sprinkle with sugar and let stand for 5 minutes. Serve warm.

COOK'S TIPS

+ *If using fresh cherries, you will need to buy about 2/3 pound (350 g) unpitted cherries.*
+ *If using a deep ovenproof dish, place it in a large roasting pan. Pour boiling water into the pan to come one-third of the way up the side of the dish, and bake until just set.*
+ *Remove the clafoutis from the oven as soon as it is set all the way through; overcooking can cause the texture to become rubbery.*

Each serving provides
184 calories, 7 g protein, 3 g fat (1 g saturated fat), 32 g carbohydrate (22 g sugars), 1 g fiber, 57 mg sodium

CHERRIES contain a high level of antioxidants such as phenols, quercetin and anthocyanins, which puts cherries in the category of "antiaging superfood." Anthocyanins, in particular, are a subject of current research into inflammatory conditions such as gout and arthritis, and due to their high anthocyanin content, cherries may protect against gout.

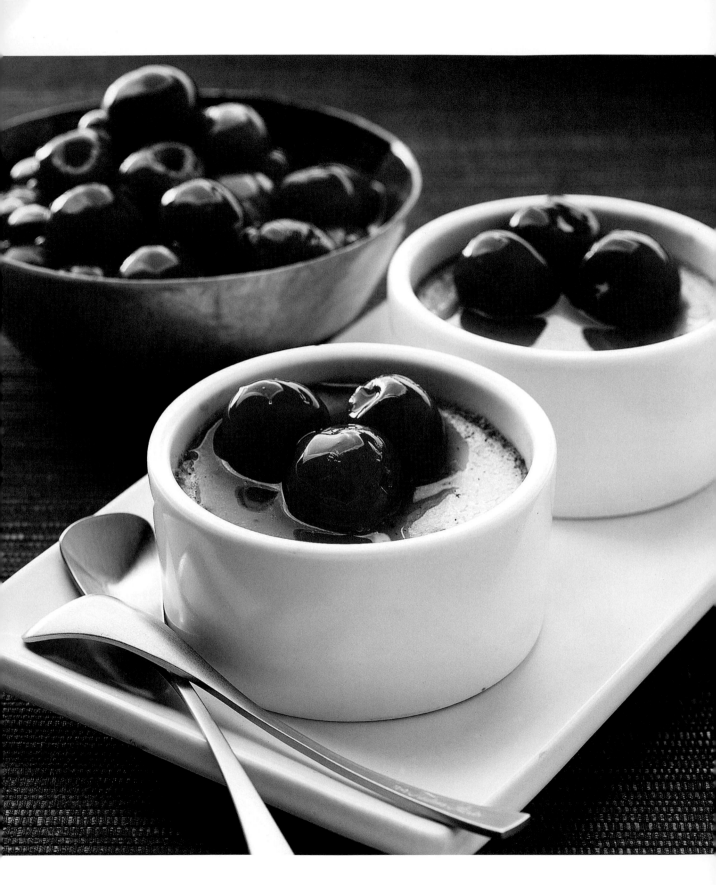

little *custard pots*

A compote of sweet–tart cherries makes the perfect accompaniment to balance the richness of these delightfully creamy custards.

SERVES 6   PREPARATION 15 MINUTES   COOKING 30 MINUTES

$2^{1}/_{2}$ cups (600 ml) low-fat milk

$^{1}/_{2}$ vanilla bean, split

2 eggs

2 egg yolks

2 tablespoons (30 ml) superfine sugar

$^{1}/_{2}$ teaspoon (2 ml) cornstarch

$1^{1}/_{2}$ tablespoons (22 ml) raw sugar

$1^{3}/_{4}$ cups (450 g) fresh cherries, pitted

2 teaspoons (10 ml) arrowroot

CHERRIES have a low GI, are rich in potassium and provide useful amounts of vitamin C.

ADDING extra egg yolks in this recipe boosts the content of vitamins A, D and E, as well as B vitamins.

1 Put the milk and vanilla bean in a saucepan over medium heat and bring just to a boil. Remove the pan from the heat, cover and set aside to infuse for 15 minutes.

2 Preheat the oven to 325°F (160°C). Put the whole eggs, egg yolks, superfine sugar and cornstarch into a heatproof bowl and lightly whisk together. Return the milk to boiling, remove the vanilla bean and slowly pour the hot milk over the egg mixture, whisking all the time. Strain the mixture into a pitcher, and pour into six $^{1}/_{2}$ cup (125 ml) ramekins or ovenproof dishes, dividing it equally among them.

3 Set the ramekins in a roasting pan or baking dish and pour in enough hot water to come halfway up the sides of the ramekins. Bake for 30–35 minutes, or until lightly set— the custards should still be slightly wobbly, as they will continue cooking for a few minutes after they are removed from the oven. Remove them from the hot water and let cool. Once cool, chill until ready to serve.

4 To make the cherry compote, put the raw sugar and $^{1}/_{2}$ cup (125 ml) water in a saucepan and heat gently until the sugar has dissolved. Bring to a boil, reduce the heat and add the cherries. Cover and simmer gently for 4–5 minutes, stirring occasionally, until tender. Remove the cherries with a slotted spoon and place in a serving bowl.

5 Mix the arrowroot with 1 tablespoon (15 ml) cold water. Stir into the cherry juices in the saucepan and simmer for 1 minute, stirring, until thickened and clear. Allow to cool for a few minutes, then pour over the cherries. Spoon some of the compote on top of each custard, and serve the rest of the compote in a bowl.

Each serving provides
180 calories, 9 g protein, 4 g fat (1 g saturated fat),
28 g carbohydrate (26 g sugars), 1 g fiber, 86 mg sodium

raspberry creams with mango & honey purée

Everyone will love this lusciously creamy yet healthy dessert made with mangoes and raspberries. This is a low-fat dessert that can be whipped up in minutes.

SERVES 4   PREPARATION
10 MINUTES   COOKING NONE

1 cup (250 g) low-fat
   Greek-style yogurt or
   low-fat cream cheese
2 tablespoons (30 ml)
   confectioners' sugar
1 large mango
1 tablespoon (15 ml) honey
1 cup (260 g) raspberries

1 Combine the yogurt and confectioners' sugar in a bowl. Slice the mango flesh from the pit, chop the flesh into chunks and purée in a blender or food processor. Stir the honey into the mango purée.

2 Set aside eight raspberries and reserve 1 tablespoon (15 ml) of the sweetened yogurt. Divide the remainder of the raspberries among four glass dishes and top with the yogurt mixture. Use a knife or the back of a spoon to create an even surface.

3 Spoon the mango purée over the yogurt. Top each portion with 1 teaspoon (5 ml) of the sweetened yogurt; garnish with raspberries.

OTHER IDEAS

+ *Use a variety of fruit instead of raspberries. Try sliced strawberries, whole blueberries, pitted cherries, halved black or green grapes, kiwi fruit, pineapple chunks or sliced bananas.*

+ *Swap the yogurt or cream cheese for ricotta, beating it thoroughly with the confectioners' sugar in step 1 until it is smooth and creamy.*

+ *Instead of mango, use peaches, nectarines or plums to make a tasty purée to complement the raspberries. Use a total of 1 1/3 cups (350 g) fruit for the purée.*

Each serving provides
170 calories, 6 g protein, 2 g fat
(1 g saturated fat), 31 g carbohydrate
(27 g sugars), 4 g fiber, 97 mg sodium

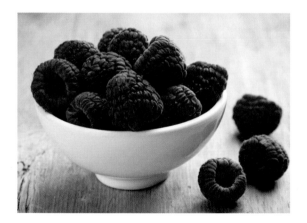

Super Food
   RASPBERRIES, like other berries, are rich in anthocyanins and ellagic acid, powerful antioxidants that help protect against cancer and heart disease.

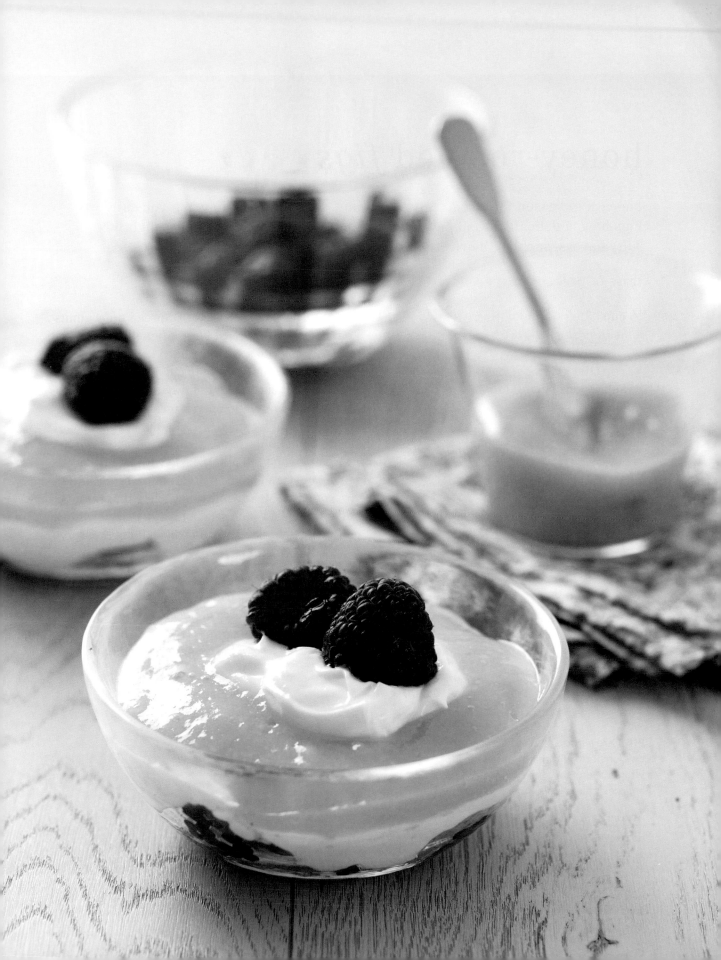

frozen strawberry mousse

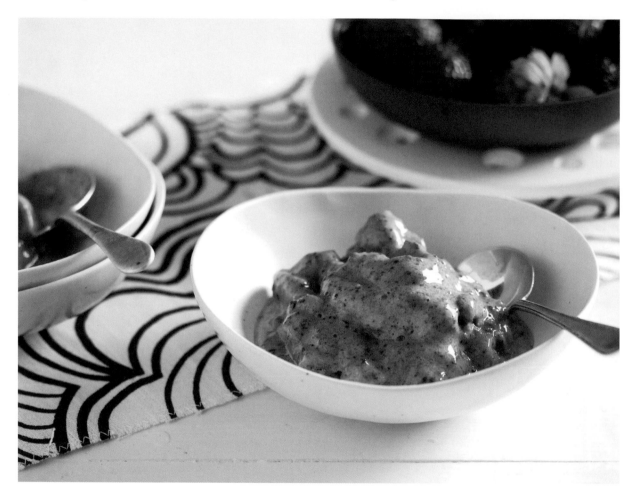

SERVES 4   PREPARATION 5 MINUTES
COOKING NONE

1 cup (250 ml) light evaporated
  milk, chilled
2 tablespoons (30 ml)
  confectioners' sugar
1 teaspoon (5 ml) grated
  orange zest
2 cups (300 g) frozen strawberries

1 Combine the chilled evaporated milk, confectioners'
  sugar and orange zest in a pitcher.
2 Put the strawberries in a food processor or blender
  and pulse until just chopped. With the motor running,
  gradually add the evaporated milk mixture and process
  until the ingredients are just combined.
3 Divide the strawberry mousse among four dessert bowls
  and serve immediately.

Each serving provides
60 calories, 3 g protein, <1 g fat (<1 g saturated fat),
11 g carbohydrate (11 g sugars), 2 g fiber, 31 mg sodium

berry whip

SERVES 2 PREPARATION 5 MINUTES
COOKING NONE

1 cup (225 g) frozen berries
²/₃ cup (150 g) frozen yogurt
2 teaspoons (10 ml)
   confectioners' sugar

1 Place the frozen berries, yogurt
and confectioners' sugar in a
blender or food processor and
blend until smooth.
2 Serve immediately in two tall
glasses or glass dishes.

OTHER IDEAS

+ *Top the berry whip with low-fat
Greek-style yogurt or fromage frais.*

+ *Serve the berry whip with crushed
ready-made meringues lightly folded
into the whip or sprinkled on top.*

+ *Here's another no-cook dessert idea
that serves 2: Pour 1 cup (250 ml)
ready-made low-fat custard into a
bowl. In a blender, purée 1 cup
(250 g) drained, canned fruit—try
cherries, apricots, peaches, plums,
mango or even fruit salad mixes. Stir
the puréed fruit into the custard.
Divide the fruit mixture between two
small glasses and chill in the freezer
for 5–15 minutes. Serve sprinkled
with toasted slivered almonds.*

Each serving provides
202 calories, 5 g protein, 5 g fat
(4 g saturated fat), 33 g carbohydrate
(28 g sugars), 5 g fiber, 49 mg sodium

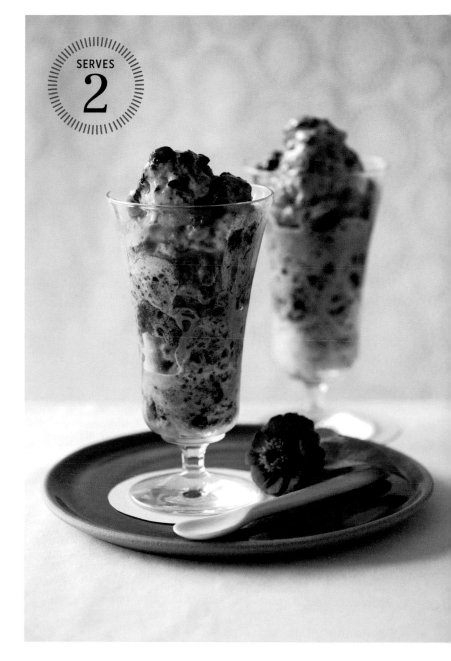

SERVES
2

index

Diabetes Cookbook

Consultant Carole Webster
Project Editor Kim Rowney
Senior Editor Samantha Kent
Project Designer Emma Ross
Senior Designer Joanne Buckley
Nutritional Analysis Toni Gumley
Proofreader Susan McCreery
Indexer Diane Harriman
Senior Production Controller Martin Milat

Diabetes Cookbook was first published in 2014 by
Reader's Digest (Australia) Pty Limited

Copyright © 2016 The Reader's Digest Association, Inc.

ISBN 978-1-62145-295-9/Epub ISBN 978-1-62145-296-6

We are committed to both the quality of our products and
the service we provide to our customers. We value your
comments, so please feel free to contact us.

> The Reader's Digest Association, Inc.
> Adult Trade Publishing
> 44 South Broadway
> White Plains, NY 10601

For more Reader's Digest products and information, visit
our website:

> www.rd.com (in the United States)
> www.readersdigest.ca (in Canada)

Diabetes Cookbook contains material previously
published in the following Reader's Digest books:
*5 Ingredient Cookbook; 30 Minute Cookbook;
Amazing Vegetables; Anti-Ageing Diet Cookbook;
Cooking for One or Two; Cooking with Herbs;
Cooking with Spices; Delicious and Healthy Food
for the Over Fifties; Desserts and Sweet Treats;
Family Favourites; Fish and Seafood; Food in a Flash;
GI Cookbook; Grandma's Quick & Thrifty Cookbook;
High Fiber Cookbook; Like Grandma Used to Make;
Low Fat No Fat Cookbook; Meat Favourites; Midweek
Meals Made Easy; Milk, Eggs and Cheese; Perfect
Pasta; Pies, Tarts and Puddings; Rice, Beans and
Grains; Super Foods Super Easy*

Printed in China

10 9 8 7 6 5 4 3 2 1